Basic Surgical Techniques

For my grandchildren

Commissioning Editor: Sue Hodgson
Project Development Manager: Kim Benson
Project Manager: Hilary Hewitt
Designer: Eric Drewery

Basic Surgical Techniques

FIFTH EDITION

R M Kirk MS FRCS

Honorary Consulting Surgeon, The Royal Free Hospital, London UK

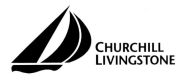

CHURCHILL
LIVINGSTONE

CHURCHILL LIVINGSTONE
An imprint of Elsevier Science Limited

First published 1973
Second edition 1978
Third edition 1989
Fourth edition 1994
Fifth edition 2002

ISBN 0 443 07122 5

British Library Cataloguing in Publication Data
A catalogue record for this book is available from the British Library

Library of Congress Cataloging in Publication Data
A catalog record for this book is available from the Library of Congress

Note
Medical knowledge is constantly changing. As new information
becomes available, changes in treatment, procedures, equipment and the
use of drugs become necessary. The authors and the publishers have
taken care to ensure that the information given in this text is accurate
and up to date. However, readers are strongly advised to confirm that
the information, especially with regard to drug usage, complies with the
latest legislation and standards of practice.

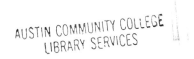
The
Publisher's
policy is to use
**paper manufactured
from sustainable forests**

Printed in China by RDC Group Limited

Contents

This is not a 'What to do' book. It aims to be a 'How to do it' book, explaining the manipulations required to carry out the individual steps that are common to most operations. It is not primarily intended to describe specific procedures but to demonstrate the fact that many of the technical skills you acquire in one area can be applied widely. However, I have used as examples the manipulative skills required for some life-saving or frequently performed procedures without trying to describe the indications, preparation, difficulties and postoperative care. These matters are discussed in *General Surgical Operations* and *Essential General Surgical Operations,* also published by Churchill Livingstone. Although I wish to describe only the practical skill aspects here, I have include enough information to place practical skills in context.

Surgery (G *cheir* = hand + *ergon* = work) is a handicraft, a creative activity, a trade as opposed to a profession. For this reason universities do not usually grant doctorates in surgery, but masterships (L *magister*, from *magnus* = great – master, shortened to Mr) signifying, among other things, a chief, a teacher, one who is eminently skilled, and instructs an apprentice (L, through French *aprendre* = to learn). Skill (Old Norse *skil* = distinction, discrimination, what is right) cannot be given to you. Some fortunate people have an inborn manipulative facility but skill is more than this – it is something you acquire by intelligent, repetitive practice, preferably under expert guidance. A refined performance is often called technique (G *techne* = art, skill) but this has two meanings – manipulative facility but also effective accomplishment; they are not synonymous, neither are they mutually exclusive. Never forget that manipulative facility does not equate with skill; skill is intelligently applied manipulation.

Much as I should like to claim it, you cannot acquire skill just by reading this book. A book can merely tell you some of the things you should do. You acquire skill by assiduously and intelligently practising the manoeuvres until they become automatic. Skills workshops allow you to perform some of the procedures under standardized conditions and, valuably, under supervision – but only a few times. Then you need to go away and practise until you can perform them perfectly, every time. A skill is an ability that is so familiar that you can accomplish a procedure automatically while concentrating on the overall circumstances, not having to concentrate on each movement. Such are our skills in driving a car, using the keyboard of a computer and playing a musical instrument.

Acquire skill in performing all the common manoeuvres, become acquainted with all the common techniques and all the equipment and instruments. They are all transferable. Many advances result from the application of a method from one area to another.

In other professions requiring skill, exponents, even at the pinnacle of achievement, accept that they require trainers and coaches. Skills are sometimes lost or bad habits develop and require to be identified and corrected. Sportsmen, musicians and airline pilots accept this but, beyond a certain point, in the past, surgeons have not accepted the need. When we are experienced we can 'get away' with imperfections but, sadly, we pass on our acquired bad habits to our trainees.

I cannot too strongly emphasize that 'doing it' is not the only important part of skill. Watch a master surgeon at work and note that before starting, he/she 'sets up' the operative field. Unnecessary articles are cleared away, the avail-ability and function of required equipment is checked, the tissues are arranged to place them in the best relationship for carrying out the next step as naturally as possible. Note that there is no frantic urgency in the progress of the operation. Everything is performed at a natural pace – each movement is an effective one; it does not require to be repeated because it was right first time.

Do not be surprised that different competent surgeons vary in their methods. Surgeons employ methods in which we believe, that serve us well. Senior surgeons become increasingly conserv-ative. As a trainee, employ the methods of your successive chiefs. In this way you will gain experience that allows you to develop your own views. You cannot improve by being inflexible. You may decide, as I have done, that it is the perfection with which procedures are performed, not the particular method, that determines success and failure. The fact that outstanding surgeons obtain better results with their methods than others may merely mean they are better surgeons. It does not *prove* that their method is the reason.

Note

The English language is a rich mixture of the Germanic, Romance and selections from the languages of all the countries with which we have had contact. Fortunately we did not have an academy that approved or condemned words attempting to enter the language. I did not have the good fortune to be educated classically and it was not until I attempted to write that I looked much into dictionaries and discovered the harvest of words and their origins. How I regret that no one explained the new vocabulary I encountered as a medical student. I once casually glanced across the page of a dictionary and discovered that the word 'parotid', which I had learned without it having any real meaning, really meant in Greek *para* = beside + *otis* = ear. I have not been able to resist the temptation to point out some of the origins of interesting words and hope you will enjoy them and start your own voyage of discovery. Many surgeons from all over the world have introduced procedures and instru-ments to which their names are attached. I have given biographical information about some of them. You have entered a wonderful, historic profession and I hope you will enjoy reading of some of the words and people associated with it.

Word origins: F, French; G, Greek; Ger, German; L, Latin; LL, Low (or Late) Latin; OE, Old English.

Apologies

Once more I apologize to women surgeons if I have written of 'he' and 'his' instead of 'he and she' and 'his and hers'. Since there is no epicene word for 'he and she', there are occasions when it is clumsy to keep repeating them. Secondly, the word 'master', in the connotation of 'expert', could not be accompanied with 'mistress,' which has quite another meaning!

I have tried in this edition to take into account left-handed surgeons by referring where possible to 'dominant' and 'non-dominant' hand.

R. M. Kirk
London, 2002

This is a 'one man' production. Because I wished to demonstrate that skills are transferable, I did not wish to make it a multi-author text. However, I have a number of distinguished colleagues, with specialized knowledge, who have generously read through chapters and advised and corrected me. Any remaining inaccuracies are mine:

Michael Brough, Consultant Plastic Surgeon, University College, Royal Free and Whittington Hospitals. London

Brian Davidson, Professor of Surgery, Royal Free Hospital, London

Deborah Eastwood, Consultant Orthopaedic Surgeon, Royal Free and Royal National Orthopaedic Hospitals, London

George Hamilton, Consultant Vascular and General Surgeon, Royal Free Hospital, London

Bryony Lovett, Consultant Colorectal Surgeon, Basildon Hospital, Essex

Adam Magos, Consultant Obstetrician and Gynaecologist, Royal Free Hospital, London.

It is a pleasure to thank the editorial and production team at Elsevier Health Sciences: Sue Hodgson, Hilary Hewitt, Kim Benson and Mick Ruddy. Thanks also go to Sukie Hunter, copyeditor and typesetter, Austin Guest, proofreader and Annette Musker, indexer.

Handling yourself

- Surgery is not a one-man/woman occupation, it is a team effort. Be a good team player.
- Keep your mental and physical state optimal. Surgery demands a balanced attitude and stamina.
- Technical skill is not acquired by attending courses – they show you what to practise and practise and practise, preferably under the expert eye of a master, until you can perform the tasks automatically.

MENTAL ATTITUDE

1. Good surgery depends on the combination of good decision-making combined with careful technical performance.

2. Carry out operations in a relaxed atmosphere of calm competence. Take each step in its correct order, complete it, check it and continue with the next one.

3. Do not allow yourself to be thrown off balance by unexpected discoveries or catastrophes.

4. In most cases your best response is to pause and assess the problem, not to rush wildly into 'doing something'.

5. It is often valuable to discuss and display the difficulty to the team. As you do so, you clarify your thoughts.

6. Panic is rare; errors more frequently result from doggedly and blindly continuing with the intended procedure instead of responding to changed circumstances.

7. A few 'characters' flourish only in an atmosphere of tension and drama. Their character is often associated with the public view of surgeons in action. It is only their present-day rarity that makes them noteworthy. Those of us to whom such tension is anathema take great care to avoid them as colleagues.

8. Never lose sight of your objectives. Particularly in emergency circumstances, avoid embarking on any unnecessary procedure.

9. Make sure that you will be able to justify your decisions to your patients, your colleagues and, more importantly, to yourself; this is especially so if you decide on a heterodox course of action.

 Key point

> Be flexible. React to changed circumstances.

PHYSICAL ATTITUDE

1. Take time to arrange the operative field so that you can carry out as much as possible in a natural manner. Do not hesitate to change the position of yourself, the patient, or a part of the patient, to facilitate your controlled accomplishment of each manoeuvre.

2. Many procedures are best performed in a particular way, such as cutting with a scalpel from away toward you and from your non-dominant to dominant side transversely. With scissors you usually cut from near to far in the sagittal plane and from dominant to non-dominant side in the transverse plane. In order to cut in an awkward direction, consider exchanging one for the other.

3. Inevitably, from time to time you must carry

out a manoeuvre in an awkward manner. Take extra care. Do not assume that 'it will be all right'.

HANDS

1. There is no ideal surgeon's hand. The shape of your hand has no bearing on your manipulative skill. However, identify the peculiarities of your own hands and fingers in order to exploit the benefits and make the best use of them. For example, the terminal phalanx, nail shape and extent of nail bed towards the tips of your fingers affect your preference for finger tip pressure or pulp pressure.

2. Your hands are important assessors of tissues. Make sure you wear the correct size of gloves and wear them correctly. Do not allow the glove fingers to project beyond yours – pull the glove fingers on fully even if this means having concertina'd wrinkles near the base of your fingers.

3. Manual dexterity and elegant performance are not the most important qualities required for success.

4. Left-handed surgeons cope well with instruments and instructions designed for right-handed people.

STABILITY

1. Surgeons do not have extraordinarily steady hands. We all have a hand tremor if we extend our arms and fingers.

2. If you hold long-handled instruments and extend them also, the tips magnify the tremor – and anxiety exaggerates this.

3. Do not feel embarrassed. Learn to control them by using a firm base as close as possible to the point of action.

4. Stand upright with arms outstretched. Now press your elbows into your sides and you find your hands are steadier. Sit, or brace your hips against a fixture to become even steadier. Rest your elbows on a table and, better, also rest the heel of your hand or use your little finger on the table (Fig. 1.1).

5. If you cannot use a base close to the active fingers, use the other hand to steady the dominant hand by grasping the wrist. If you need to reach to make an action – for example when you are cutting ligatures as an assistant – use the fingers of the

inactive hand on which to rest the scissors (Fig. 1.2). If no other base exists, place the 'heels' of your hands together when carrying out a manoeuvre such as threading a needle (Fig. 1.3).

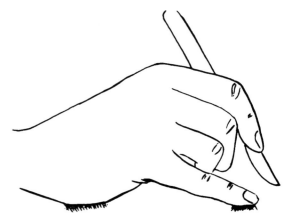

Fig. 1.1 Your wrist and little finger rest on the base, forming a steadying bridge while you hold a scalpel to make a precision incision.

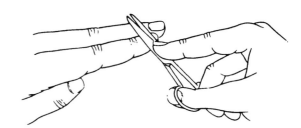

Fig. 1.2 Steady an instrument by resting it on the fingers of the other hand.

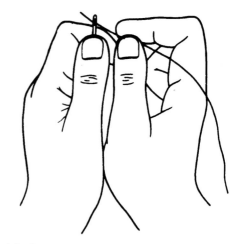

Fig. 1.3 Press your wrists together while threading a needle.

6. If you need to carry out a smooth movement, try practising it in the air first, as a golfer does before making a stroke.

TECHNIQUE

1. There are two meanings to the word (G *techne* = art, skill). 'Good technique' is often used in admiration of, for example, a surgeon's or a musician's graceful and elegant performance. The second, more important, meaning is the perfect accomplishment of a task. The two meanings are not mutually exclusive.

2. Good technique demands concentration and practice. The famous and successful golfer Gary Player is reported to have brought off a difficult shot. A spectator called out, 'That was lucky, Gary,' and he replied, 'Yes, the more I practise and the harder I try, the luckier I get.'

Key point

- Surgeons with natural talent are not always as successful as less gifted surgeons, because they do not think they need to make such an effort. However good or mediocre you are, make the most of your abilities by trying hard and practising to improve your performance.

3. In the past, trainee surgeons spent many hours in the operating theatre, repeatedly practising our craft. We were rarely supervised and therefore often accumulated bad habits – and in turn passed them on to our trainees. Do not consider supervision as unnecessary. Take every opportunity to learn from masters by assisting them, by asking them to watch and correct you. Sportsmen and women and musicians at the pinnacle of their careers, and airline pilots, do not feel demeaned by having coaches, tutors or inspectors to improve their performance and check them to correct acquired bad habits.

4. Acquire *coordinated pattern skills*. Those of us who drive cars remember the initial difficulties of using our hands to manipulate many controls, our two feet to coordinate with three pedals for a manual gearbox, our eyes to look ahead, to the sides and into the rear view mirrors, and our ears to register warning sounds. As we concentrated on one aspect, others caused problems. Everything had to be managed from a cerebral, conscious level. We now get into our cars and without any effort, extend our awareness of 'body size' to the volume of the car. We merely make a conscious decision to 'Drive' and make the combination of controlled actions that result in us starting the car, watching for a gap in the traffic and driving off without having to think what we are doing. The control is semi-automatic, from the cerebellum and other centres.

You acquired the skill by practising until you did not have to think about it, yet did it skilfully. Practise surgical manoeuvres in the same assiduous repetitive manner to hone your operative skills. Manipulate instruments so they become natural extensions of your hands, tie knots until you accomplish perfect ones automatically, in whatever position you start and whichever hand is the most active. You may still identify aspiring surgeons tying knots on the buttons of their white coats, or with their hands in their pockets practising how to apply and release haemostatic forceps with either hand. You can practise inserting sutures using any material and any thread, provided you can beg or borrow the instruments and sutures.

You will recognize when you have acquired a skill – try demonstrating it to someone else, or try carrying it out in a hurry. In each case you will become clumsy, because you have 'brought' the control up to your conscious brain!

5. Exploit your acquired skills so that they release you to concentrate on the vital assessment and decision-making aspects of the operation.

Key points

- Learn what to do from books, courses and especially from watching masters.
- Convert what you have learned into a skill by conscientious and critical repetition until it is automatic.
- From time to time check, or have checked, that you have not relapsed into bad habits.
- Do not rush – it strips you of your skill. Do things once, correctly.

ASSISTING AT OPERATIONS

1. A single-handed operator cannot always carry out several tasks simultaneously. A good assistant can facilitate the operation.

2. Do not miss an opportunity to assist at operations. Do not look upon it as a necessary boring prelude to carrying out the procedure yourself. The privilege of assisting a skilled operator allows you to acquire judgement and technique both consciously and unconsciously, so that, when you come to perform the procedure yourself, you will automatically adopt safe and effective techniques.

3. Make an opportunity to read up the anatomy and pathology that will be important. This will enormously increase the value you will gain from assisting at the operation.

4. Most surgeons acquire skill and safe techniques without being aware of them, and therefore they fail to draw their assistants' attention to them. Observe every manoeuvre and at opportune moments enquire if you do not understand the reason for it.

5. Note that the surgeon performs some manoeuvres in a routine, relaxed fashion, while taking extreme care over others. Make sure you know why.

6. Notice that good surgeons keep the operative field tidy.

Key point

- When the surgeon is not directly performing part of the operation, consider very carefully why. The likelihood is that he or she is assessing the situation or 'setting up' the equipment, lighting, exposure, and the tissues, to make the next step a standardized, routine action. When you become the operator, remember to perform these two vital activities. They mark out an expert.

---

7. As you are asked to assist, try to anticipate what is required without seeming to attempt to take over the operation. Be sensitive to the atmosphere. The surgeon may be relaxed during routine parts but require quietness in order to concentrate on difficult or crucial parts. If you are asked your opinion, give it quietly and honestly. If you think you have seen something the surgeon has missed or you think a mistake is about to be made, say so. If your warning has been heard but there is no change of action, recognize that it is the surgeon's responsibility. Do not indulge in argument. Afterwards, at an opportune moment, discuss the matter to improve your understanding.

8. Do not be disloyal to the surgeon. You may think an error has been made, or that the surgeon is incompetent. If you are confident of your facts, you should at the right time express them. However, unless you are sure, you may later, with increasing maturity, modify your former judgements, and blush with shame over some of them. The commonest fault of inexperienced young surgeons is to be dazzled by technical brilliance and remain as yet unaware of the more important judgements that have to be made. They are rarely black and white – more usually they are shades of grey – and the particular shade is contentious.

9. If you are fortunate enough to be delegated part of the operation, in your enthusiasm to impress the surgeon do not choose to display your operative speed. Rather, concentrate on being calm and careful. Prepare yourself by acquiring the simple skills of knot tying, handling of the tissues and instruments, and safe dissection. It is intensely irritating to be inveigled into delegating part of the operation only to find that simple competencies have not been mastered.

10. As you become more competent and as you are given more personal responsibility you will learn even more from assisting than formerly, since you will be aware of more of the problems. You may then be awarded the privileged relationship with the surgeon of being treated on equal terms while you both discuss and demonstrate the finer points of operative surgery. You will, when you are a fully competent surgeon, realize how much it is appreciated to be able to discuss problems with an intelligent and thoughtful assistant. The solution that is mutually arrived at will be a source of satisfaction and a lesson for the future if it proves correct, and the arguments that led to it will be a solace if it proves unsuccessful.

Handling instruments

Scalpel
Scissors
Dissecting forceps (thumb forceps)
Artery forceps (haemostatic forceps,
    haemostats)
Tissue forceps
Needle-holders
Retractors
Clamps
Mechanical devices

- Modern instruments have reached a high degree of perfection. Treat them with respect.
- Learn to handle and become familiar with standard instruments, since they are surgical extensions of your hands.
- Do not pass instruments from hand to hand. Invariably keep and pass sharp instruments in kidney dishes to avoid the risks of acquiring, or passing on, infection including viral diseases.

SCALPEL

1. The scalpel (L *scalpere* = to cut) is the traditional instrument of surgeons. Solid, reusable knives are still used for cutting tough tissues, but some instruments are totally disposable.

2. If you use a scalpel with a disposable blade, fit and remove the blade while holding it clear of the sharp edge with forceps, not with fingers. If it slips you will avoid sustaining a cut.

3. Use a scalpel for making deliberate cuts into tissues, dividing them with the minimum trauma in order to cut skin, separate tissues to reach a targeted area, divide and resect tissues.

4. In order to limit damage, draw the belly of the blade across the target rather than exerting excessive pressure that may result in an uncontrolled cut. Draw the knife blade under controlled pressure to determine the depth of cut.

5. For cutting skin and similar structures, hold the knife in a manner similar to that for holding a table knife. Keep the knife horizontal, suspended below your pronated hand, held between thumb and middle finger. Place your index finger on the back of the knife at the base of the blade, to control the pressure exerted on it. Wrap your ring and little fingers around the handle to reinforce your steadying grip, while the end of the handle rests against the hypothenar eminence (Fig. 2.1).

6. When you need to produce a small puncture or a short, precise incision, or cut a fine structure, hold the knife like a pen (see Fig. 1.1).

7. As a rule you cut in the sagittal plane from far to near, and in the transverse plane from non-dominant to dominant side. If you need to cut from dominant to non-dominant side, consider going to the other side of the operating table, using your non-dominant hand or using scissors.

8. Do not misuse the scalpel by attempting to cut

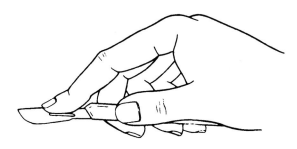

Fig. 2.1 Holding the scalpel for cutting skin. Draw the belly of the knife, not the point, across the skin.

metal or bone, or try to lever the knife during a cutting manoeuvre. Do not continue to use a blunt scalpel since, once the sharp edge is lost, you need to apply excessive pressure and the incision is uneven.

9. Never make a casual incision without first assessing the exact situation; some are irretrievable. Before making a critical incision plan it and if necessary first draw an intended line on the skin with Bonney's blue ink. Occasionally it is worth practising in the air before making a smooth, controlled cut, as golfers do when preparing to make a putt. If an important structure will be endangered, interpose a protective instrument such as a retractor. When you are about to cut a linear structure in the depths you may be able to place a grooved dissector beneath it, to protect deeper tissues.

A special scalpel exists, called a bistoury, conjectured to be named after Pistorium (modern Pistoja) in Tuscany where they were made. It has a long, thin, curved blade, blunt-ended for side cutting, sharp tipped for end cutting through a small opening. I have never used one, preferring to improve the access and cut under direct vision.

SCISSORS

1. The cutting action of scissors (LL *cisorium* = a cutting instrument, from *caedere* = to cut) results from the moving-edge contact between the blades, which are given a slight set towards each other. If the blades spring apart, the cutting action is replaced by a chewing effect. The blades may be forced apart if delicate scissors are used to cut tough tissues.

2. Scissors are made for right-handed users and the lateral pressure of the right-handed thumb tends to result in the blades being pressed together. When held in the left hand the pressure of the thumb tends to lever the blades apart.

3. Most surgical scissors have round tips but for special purposes pointed blades may be used. The blades may be straight, curved or angled.

4. With your hand in mid-pronation, hold scissors by inserting only part of the first phalanx of the thumb through one ring (called a 'bow' by the manufacturers); this controls the moving blade. Insert only the first phalanx of the ring finger into the other ring, and

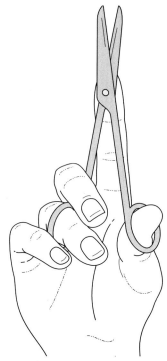

Fig. 2.2 Holding scissors. Insert only half the first phalanx of your thumb and all the first phalanx of the ring finger into the rings. Wrap your middle and little fingers around the ring finger. Place your index finger on the hinge.

wrap the middle and little fingers around the handle to steady it; this will be the fixed blade (Fig. 2.2). Place the tip of your index finger on the hinge.

5. Hold your hand in mid-pronation. If you are right-handed and you press with your thumb towards the left while opening and closing the scissors, note that the blades bind together. If you hold the scissors in your left hand in mid-pronation and press with your thumb towards the right, the binding effect is reduced between the blades – and abolished if the joint is loose.

 Key point

- If you are left-handed, using scissors to make a crucial cut, insert the whole terminal phalanx of your thumb through its ring so you can flex it at the interphalangeal joint and draw the ring to your left to increase the binding force between the blades.

6. As a rule your hand is most comfortable in the mid-prone position but if you are cutting down a deep hole try fully supinating your hand so that you have a clearer view of the structures at the tip. A hand in pronation may obstruct your view.

7. Choose the correct scissors for the task. Mayo's are excellent all-purpose scissors (from the celebrated Clinic of the brothers William, born 1861, and Charles, born 1865, both died 1939, came well-'designed scissors and needle-holder). The tips are rounded, the blades do not spring apart, so they cut cleanly. Use lighter scissors for very light work only. Remember that it is more difficult to make the blades of curved scissors accurately engage along their whole length. If you are cutting down a hole, prefer long-handled scissors so that the rings remain outside the hole. The longer the scissors, the more likely is any tremor to be magnified, so be willing to rest the hinge on the fingers of your non-dominant hand.

8. It is fortunate that scalpel and scissors cut in opposite directions. Scissors cut in the sagittal plane from near to far but, when you need to cut from far to near, it may be practical to use a scalpel. In the transverse plane scissors cut most conveniently from dominant towards the non-dominant side. When you need to cut in the transverse plane from your non-dominant side towards your dominant side, consider moving to the other side of the operating table or using a scalpel. If you are reasonably ambidextrous, change the scissors to your non-dominant hand; alternatively, swing the scissors round in your dominant hand, so they point towards your elbow (Fig. 2.3).

9. For rather snobbish reasons, scissors are despised as a dissecting instrument by some, who consider that tissues should never be divided except with a scalpel. I must admit that some surgeons are a delight to watch, wielding a scalpel with great skill and effectiveness. However, appearance is not all. I have also admired surgeons using scissors with great versatility, inserting the tips into a tissue plane, gently opening the blades to create a defined bridge of tissue, withdrawing the scissors, inserting one blade beneath, one blade superficial to the bridge and dividing it, proceeding in a rapid, effective manner, without the need to change instruments.

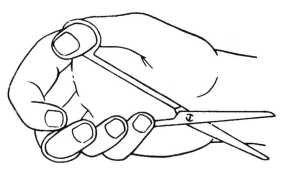

Fig. 2.3 Cutting from left to right while holding scissors in the right hand.

Watch others, try both methods, make up your own mind. I suspect that you will conclude, like me, that there is room for both techniques.

DISSECTING FORCEPS (THUMB FORCEPS)

1. It is not clear whether the word derived from *ferriceps* (L *ferrum* = iron + *capere* = to take), or from *formus* (L = hot + *capere*). Forceps grip when compressed between thumb and fingers. When released the blades separate because they are made of springy steel and are given a set during manufacture. Dissecting forceps form an excellent multipurpose instrument. As a rule, hold them like a pen in your non-dominant hand, since you usually have another instrument in your dominant hand (Fig. 2.4). They do not usually have a locking mechanism because they

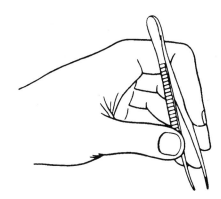

Fig. 2.4 Gripping dissecting forceps. As a rule, hold them in the non-dominant hand, since the dominant hand usually holds another instrument.

are intended to provide only a temporary grip; indeed, avoid grasping tissue at one point, or applying traction for a prolonged period or you will damage it.

2. The commonest types are toothed and non-toothed but various shaped tips are available, such as rings for grasping soft viscera. Delicate forceps have a post on the inside of one blade that engages with a hole in the other blade, to ensure that the tips meet accurately.

3. They may be extremely delicate for use during microsurgery or be large and strong for grasping tough tissues.

4. Toothed forceps have at least one tooth on one tip, interdigitating with two teeth on the opposing tip. The intention is that the teeth puncture the surface of the tissue, tethering it and so preventing it from slipping, rather than holding it by strong compression, which may be more damaging. Skin is tolerant of punctures but is severely injured by crushing, so toothed forceps are usually employed to grasp it. Very tough, slippery tissues such as fascia, fibrocartilage and bone are best grasped with toothed forceps.

5. Non-toothed forceps exert their grip through serrations on the opposing tips. Use them when manipulating blood vessels, bowel and small ducts, since punctures of these cause leakage. Provided the closed tips are used to act as counterpressure and manipulate it, rather than to grip it, they are suitable for use on skin.

6. Learn to palm forceps (Fig. 2.5), retaining them with your ring and little fingers, to free the dominant fingers and thumb, while tying knots.

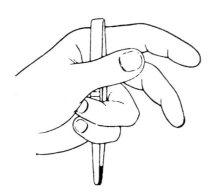

Fig. 2.5 Learn to palm dissecting forceps, freeing your active fingers to hold tissues or instruments and to tie knots.

7. The closed blades of round-nosed non-toothed forceps make an excellent dissecting tool. Insert them in the desired plane and allow their springiness to open up the tissues gently. Sometimes you can push them along, to act as a wedge, separating fragile tissues in a plane of cleavage; you can then insert the deep blade of slightly opened scissors running in the gap between the forceps blades to cut the overlying tissues, or use a scalpel, while the deeper tissues are protected from injury. This method is valuable when displaying a longitudinal structure such as a blood vessel, nerve or tendon.

ARTERY FORCEPS (HAEMOSTATIC FORCEPS, HAEMOSTATS)

1. Haemostatic forceps (G *haema* = blood + *stasis* = stoppage) were devised by the great French surgeon Ambroise Paré (1510–1590) with a scissors action and were improved, by the addition of a ratchet so they could be locked, by Sir Thomas Spencer Wells (1818–1897) after whom they are often named. Note that the tips alone meet when they are lightly closed; the proximal parts of the blades are slightly separated. The basic design is so versatile that it has been adapted from fine 'mosquito' forceps to heavy, toothed grasping forceps. When the handles are compressed, the ratchets lock. To release them you need to compress them lightly to overcome the slight overhang of the ratchet, separate the handles in a plane at right angles to the hinge action, and open the handles. Practise the action so that you can skilfully and controllably apply and remove them automatically.

2. Because these forceps can be applied and left in place, always ensure that the shafts are sufficiently long so that the handles remain outside the wound. Short-handled forceps left in the wound are easily forgotten, so always check the number at the end of the procedure.

3. Insert the first phalanx only of your thumb and of your ring finger into the rings of the opened forceps, with your index finger on the hinge (Fig. 2.6) Grasp small vessels near the tips of the forceps but always leave the point protruding; a single click of the ratchet may suffice. Grasp thicker vessels nearer the

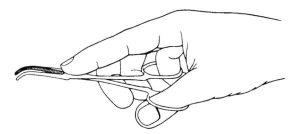

Fig. 2.6 Holding artery forceps. Notice that these are curved. When capturing fine bleeding points you may hold them with the tips pointing down but when capturing substantial vessels, apply them with the concavity of the blades uppermost.

hinge where there is a gap between the blades, to avoid straining the forceps. Apply curved forceps on to substantial vessels with the concavity uppermost and tips extending just beyond the vessel, to retain the ligature that will be tied beneath the forceps.

 Key point

- Avoid picking up extraneous tissue. If you apply a ligature around it and the vessel, the attachment will anchor the ligature and allow the vessel, as it retracts, to withdraw from it and rebleed.

4. If you are the assistant, you will be expected to remove the forceps when the vessel is ligated (see p. 33). The surgeon will either expect you to lift the handle of the forceps to allow the end of the ligature to be passed from hand to hand on your side of the vessel, or will stretch the ligature between two hands on your side of the vessel while you reach over it to grasp the handles of the forceps. Gently lower the handles of curved forceps while the ligature passes under the projecting point of the haemostat to encircle the vessel only. When the first half-hitch is formed and tightened, you should, in a controlled manner, release and remove the haemostat. Ideally, remove it with your left hand if you are right-handed, since you will hold scissors in your dominant hand, ready to cut the ligature. Reach for one ring between your index finger and thumb; this is to be the static ring. Insert part of the first phalanx

of the ring finger in the other ring and steady it by pressure from outside the ring, with the little finger (Fig. 2.7). Gently compress the rings together to release the overlap of the ratchet, lever the handles in opposite directions at right angles to the joint and gently open the forceps without pulling them off. When the final half hitch has been tightened the surgeon will hold up the ends of the ligature while you cut them, using the scissors held in the right hand.

 Key points

- When an important vessel is being tied you may be asked to gently slacken the forceps while a first ligature is being tied and tightened; then re-clamp the forceps while a second ligature is tied and tightened, then remove the forceps.
- If the ligature is faulty, if it has encircled the tips of the forceps – and will, therefore, fall off when you remove the forceps – do not remove them but warn the surgeon.

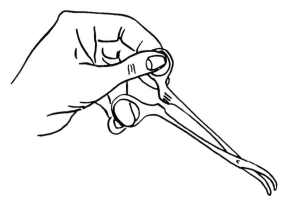

Fig. 2.7 Removing artery forceps with the left hand.

TISSUE FORCEPS

1. These rely for their grip on the shape and the apposing surfaces of their blades in contact with the tissues to grasp them but not damage them. Some encircle the tissues, some have large ring blades through which the tissues bulge, or rough surfaces, or teeth (Fig. 2.8).

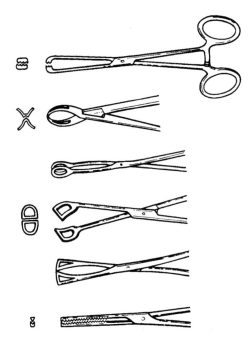

Fig. 2.8 Tissue forceps. From above downwards: Allis, Lane's, ring, Babcock's, Duval and Kocher's toothed forceps.

2. Use them in circumstances when traction sutures or a sharp hook may cut out, when the tissues are too slippery to be held with smooth retractors, and when the direction of traction needs to be varied. Do not neglect to make use of gravity, tapes, packing, or extending the incision to avoid damage caused by applying traction with metal forceps.

3. If you need to apply strong traction of tough tissues, use forceps with a powerful grip rather than inadequate forceps that are likely to pull off, tearing the tissues and straining the forceps. When the tissues are fragile, use delicate forceps, apply them carefully, do not drag on them and remove them as soon as possible. Several lightweight forceps may give a better grip and do less damage than a single pair of heavy forceps.

NEEDLE-HOLDERS

1. In the past many surgeons held needles in our hands. The risk of sustaining or transmitting infection, especially viral diseases, has made the practice unsustainable. Needles should not come into contact with your skin but should always be held with a needle-holder. Most needles are now curved but use the needle-holder to drive all types of needle through the tissues.

2. There is a great variety of needle-holders but a relatively few are in common use (Fig. 2.9). They grip the needle with specially designed jaws. Most of them are straight and are designed to be rotated in their long axis with a pronation/supination action of the hand to drive the needle through the tissues in a curved path.

3. Mayo's is the simplest model, used in many modifications, similar in design to haemostatic forceps, with ratchet closure and controlled in the same manner. Sir Harold Gillies (1882–1960), the New-Zealand-born father of British plastic surgery, invented a non-locking combined needle-holder and scissors. Ophthalmic surgeons use a small holder for the fine stitching required.

4. Grip the curved needle between the jaws of the needle-holder. The needle makes a right angle with the holder. Have the needle point facing towards your non-dominant side and pointing upwards when your hand is in the mid-prone position, because you more easily drive the needle through by starting with your hand fully pronated, progressively supinating.

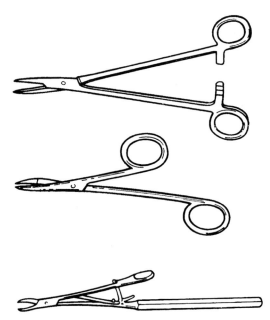

Fig. 2.9 Needle-holders. From above downwards: Mayo's, Gillies's combined needle-holder and scissors, and fine ophthalmic needle-holder.

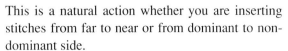

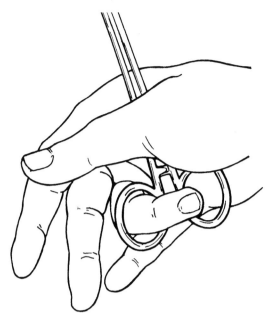

Fig. 2.10 Palm the needle-holder by removing your thumb from one ring and rotate the instrument so that it lies in the interspace between the thumb and the second metacarpal. It slightly restricts movement of the thumb.

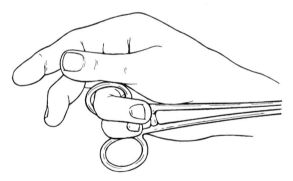

Fig. 2.11 Palm the needle-holder so that it points towards your elbow and flex your little finger between the rings. Your thumb is completely free.

Fig. 2.12 To reverse the direction of the needle, rotate the needle in the needle-holder, then merely rotate the needle-holder through 180°. This manoeuvre has been popularised by Mr W.E.G. Thomas.

This is a natural action whether you are inserting stitches from far to near or from dominant to non-dominant side.

5. If you are stitching in the depths of a wound, use a long-handled needle-holder, otherwise your hand is inside the entrance, blocking your view.

6. When you are inserting and tying stitches, or need to carry out some other short action, it is very convenient to palm the needle-holder. Remove your thumb from one ring, retaining your ring finger in the other. Swing the shaft of the needle-holder into the first interspace between the thumb and second metacarpal (Fig. 2.10) or swing it until it points back towards your elbow and flex your little finger into the space between the rings to retain it (Fig. 2.11). Do not retain the needle in the holder if you intend to palm it.

7. Occasionally you need to stitch alternately from right to left and then left to right, or far to near then near to far. In order to avoid the need to remove and replace the needle, merely turn it in the needle-holder, then turn the needle-holder through 180° in its long axis and gain a fresh grip (Fig. 2.12).

RETRACTORS

These are extremely useful when you wish to display and carry out a procedure on a deeply placed organ. Some are hand-held, some are self-retaining (Fig. 2.13). Use them carefully so you do not damage structures inadvertently. Ask your assistant who is retracting for you to use minimal traction and to relax it whenever it is unnecessary. Sometimes a change of approach, retraction by a hand placed over a pack, is less damaging than a metal retractor.

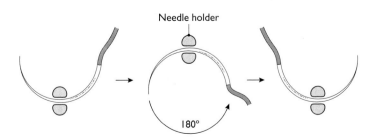

Needle holder

180°

CLAMPS

1. A wide variety of clamps has been devised to fulfil the differing needs of grasping, joining and compressing structures (Fig. 2.14), and the mechanisms for fixing them vary from spring handles to ratchets, locking hinges and screws.

2. As opposed to haemostatic forceps, which are intended to clamp blood vessels that will be permanently sealed, bulldog clips and Potts's artery clamps are designed to occlude them temporarily without damaging them.

3. In order to prevent leakage of contaminating contents from the bowel, control oozing from the cut edges and steady the ends while carrying out an anastomosis, many surgeons apply non-crushing clamps near the ends, including the vessels in the mesentery. In some models, the clamps on each side of the anastomosis can be fixed together. Other surgeons condemn the use of bowel clamps. Make up your own mind.

If you do apply them across the mesentery, make sure you apply them very lightly, or just firmly enough to occlude the arteries. Do not merely occlude the veins while leaving the arteries patent. If you do so, the bowel and the occluded veins in the mesentery will become congested and may rupture, bleed into the mesentery and be difficult to identify.

4. When you resect bowel you may place two crushing clamps side by side at each point of division and cut between them. In this way the cut ends are sealed. If you then intend to join the bowel ends do not fail to excise the crushed, sealed strip to expose the lumen.

MECHANICAL DEVICES

These are sometimes valuable to save time and to facilitate difficult manoeuvres. Do not overuse them or become dependent on them, because traditional methods are, overall, more versatile.

Haemostatic clips

1. Metal clips fit into the jaws of special forceps and can be applied across blood vessels and ducts to occlude them. The clips are cleverly designed so that

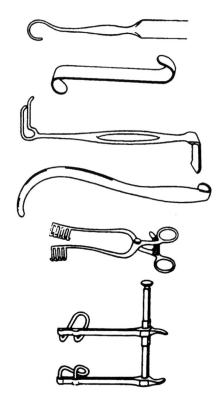

Fig. 2.13 Retractors. From above downwards: hook, malleable copper, Czerny, Deaver, self-retaining and Gosset self-retaining.

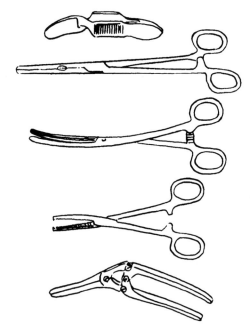

Fig. 2.14 Clamps. Above, three non-crushing clamps: 'bulldog', Potts arterial and intestinal. Below, two crushing clamps: Kocher's arterial and Payr's lever-action intestinal.

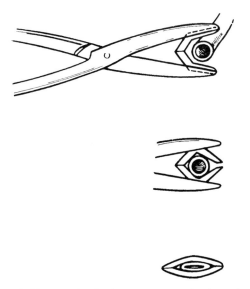

Fig. 2.15 Vascular clip. As you compress the clamp, the clip first closes around the vessel or duct and then compresses and occludes it

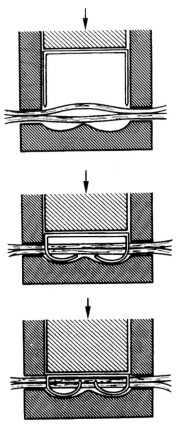

when they are closed their tips meet first so that the tubular structure does not slip away (Fig. 2.15). Further compression occludes the lumen. Some instruments apply a series of clips from a mechanical or powered applicator. Another instrument applies two clips across a structure while cutting between them with a single action. Haemostatic clips are useful as radio-opaque markers to help identify their position after operation. They can be placed at intervals around a tumour in order to plan radiotherapy, and to estimate subsequent shrinkage as a result of treatment. A disadvantage of clips compared with ligatures and sutures is that they catch on hands, instruments and swabs and can be pulled off.

2. Biodegradable clips are available as an alternative to metal clips. They are slowly absorbed.

Stapling devices

1. The principle of mechanical staplers in surgery is exactly the same as paper stapling machines. An inverted-U-shaped staple is driven through the target tissues and then hits a shaped anvil that turns the ends (Fig. 2.16). The tissues should not be crushed because the ends are so turned as to form the shape of the letter 'B' lying on its face.

Fig. 2.16 The principles of stapling action. As you close the instrument you drive the staple points through the two layers of tissue which then hit the anvil and are turned over to form the shape of a B lying on its face.

2. Modern straight staplers apply two offset parallel lines of staples. One type applies four parallel lines and at the same time cuts along the centre to produce a double line of staples on each side of the cut. This can be used to produce a stoma between two segments of bowel. Insert the staple magazine containing the staples into one bowel lumen through a stab wound, the anvil bar into the other bowel lumen through a stab wound; lock the two limbs together and actuate the instrument. When you unlock and remove the two limbs there remain only the two stab wounds to close, leaving a side-to-side anastomosis.

3. Circular staplers (Fig. 2.17) produce an end-to-end anastomosis. There are two concentric offset rows of staples in the magazine head. At the end of a spindle is a removable circular anvil. In order to

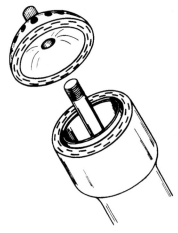

Fig. 2.17 The head of a circular stapling device. Two offset concentric rings of staples are set into the magazine below and to the right. The anvil head lies above and to the left. The anvil is attached to the spindle and can be screwed down on to the magazine.

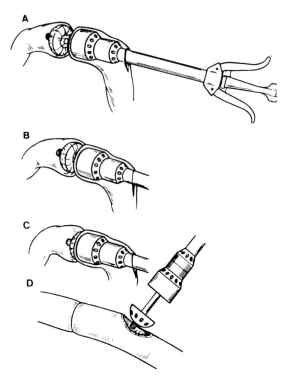

Fig. 2.18 End-to-end union of bowel. **A** Insert the staple head into the bowel through a side incision, pass it through the end and into the segment to be joined on. **B** Insert purse-string sutures round both bowel ends and tie them to draw a ring of each end of bowel into the gap between the magazine and anvil. **C** Close the gap so that the two inturned ends are brought into contact. Now actuate the instrument to staple the bowel ends together and cut off the internal fringes of bowel. **D** After separating the anvil from the empty magazine, withdraw the head of the instrument and then close the entry hole.

form an anastomosis, insert the staple head through a side hole in the bowel wall, or, when performing a low colorectal anastomosis, for example, insert it through the anus. Fix the anvil on the end of the spindle, and introduce it into the other end of bowel (Fig. 2.18). Insert a purse-string suture around each bowel end and tighten and tie them. This draws one end over the staple magazine end, the other over the anvil head. The anvil can now be screwed down to trap the two inverted bowel ends between the staple heads, without crushing them. Now activate the instrument. The staples are thrust through both layers of inverted bowel ends, hit the anvil and are turned over. Simultaneously, an inner circular knife is pushed through to cut off the excess inverted bowel ends. Now separate the anvil from staple head and gently withdraw the instrument with a twisting motion. Examine the trimmed ends encircling the central spindle. They should be complete toroids – 'doughnuts,' confirming that the anastomosis has been perfectly carried out through the whole circumference. Check the circumference externally. If you created a side hole to insert the instrument, close it.

Skin staplers

1. Skin staplers must be inserted without the presence of an anvil to turn them (Fig. 2.19). The central section of the U-shaped staple is held while the outer ends are pushed through the skin and then bent so that the ends meet, forming a closed ring.

2. They are removed by straightening the base of the 'U' to open out the ends so that the staples can be withdrawn.

3. Staples can be inserted from a magazine containing a number for ease. The former clips devised by Gaston Michel of Nancy in France (1875–1937) have been virtually abandoned.

4. Although there are occasions when staples are valuable in allowing rapid closure, concentrate on acquiring skill in stitching, which is nearly as quick and can be used in almost any situation.

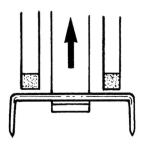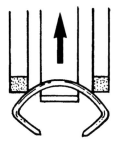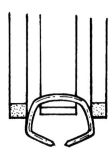

Fig. 2.19 The principle of skin staplers. Since there is no anvil beneath the skin, the staples must be formed from without. The sequence of action proceeds from left to right. The central column of the stapler has a lip beneath the middle section of the staple to hold it, while the outer pillars descend to bend the staple, creating a closed ring.

3

Handling threads

with Bryony Lovett

- Threads of various materials are used extensively for ligating (binding) and suturing (sewing).
- Manufacturers strive to produce threads that are strong, reliable, produce minimal inflammatory, allergic or carcinogenic response. In some cases the threads are coated to improve the surface characteristics. Most threads are sterilized by gamma rays and presented in sealed packets.
- All foreign materials inserted into the body evoke a reaction but some are relatively inert. Natural products tend to evoke an inflammatory reaction, stimulating manufacturers to produce synthetic (G *syn* = together + *thesis* = a placing; hence, putting together) materials that are less reactive.
- Threads may be absorbable, such as catgut, which is no longer used, and some synthetics. Non-absorbable threads include silk, nylon and other synthetics. Most 'non-absorbables' are changed within the tissues.

THREAD CHARACTERISTICS

1. Catgut, prepared from twisted strips of the collagenous submucosal coat of sheep or cow's intestine, loses its strength and is absorbed capriciously by means of the inflammatory response. If it is denatured with chromic acid, it is absorbed more slowly. It is no longer used because of the potential risks of transmitting bovine spongiform encephalopathy (BSE).

2. Excellent synthetic absorbables are stronger, evoke little reaction and are absorbed predictably. Some slowly absorbed materials retain strength for long enough to replace non-absorbable threads in certain circumstances.

3. Monofilament substances include polydioxanone (PDS®), polyglyconate (Maxon®) and glycomer 631 (Biosin®). Monofilaments, since they expose less surface to the body tissues, cause less reaction than do multifilaments and are preferable in the presence of infection because their smooth surfaces, produced by extrusion, do not provide a nidus for microorganisms. Against this they are often difficult to handle and, because they have smooth surfaces, knots do not hold so well. If the smooth surface is damaged the threads are seriously weakened.

4. Multifilament substances include polyglactin 910 (Vicryl®), polyglycolic acid (Dexon®), and lactomer 9–1 (Polysorb®). They handle excellently, tie well and retain their strength for prolonged periods. Do not pull them roughly through the tissues: their surfaces are not as smooth as monofilaments, so there is a dragging and sawing effect.

5. Non-absorbable sutures include silk and linen, which knot easily and reliably. Polyesters, polypropylene and polyamides are synthetics and evoke minimal tissue reaction. Monofilament forms are strong but are smooth and do not form strong knots. They have 'memory' and tend to return to the straight form in which they were extruded. Like monofilament absorbables, the smooth-surfaced

monofilament non-absorbables are seriously weakened if this surface is damaged, rather like a glass surface that has been scored. Multifilament forms handle well and knot well. Stainless steel causes almost no tissue reaction but is difficult to handle; have your assistant guide the loops of wire to avoid snags and twists.

 Key point

- Do not use excessive force when pulling on a thread. You may break it but at least you are aware of this. Worse, you may weaken it and it will break later. Do not weaken the thread by dragging it over sharp edges, or roughly scraping the strands together when tightening knots. Do not grasp threads with metal instruments except in sections that you will excise.

6. Twisted threads have a 'lay'; twist them one way and you tighten the twist and compact the thread, twist it the other way and you unlay the thread fibres. Twist monofilament or braided threads either way and there is no difference in behaviour. If you twist a slack thread it forms a loop (Fig. 3.1). When you form a loose loop in a thread you must give it a twist or it will unwind. This is especially so in heavier cords; watch a seaman coiling a heavy rope.

7. Threads have an almost fiendish propensity to catch around the handles of surgical instruments or any other projection. Whenever you are handling threads arrange them so that they do not catch, remove all unnecessary instruments from the area, or cover the projections with towels to protect them.

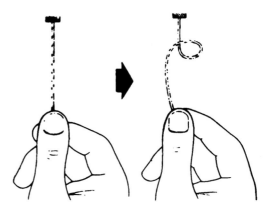

Fig. 3.1 Effect of twisting a thread.

 Key point

- Surgeons vary in their choice of threads. Note and use those chosen by your chief. Make up your own mind so that at the completion of training you will have experienced a range of materials and can make a sensible choice.

THREAD SIZES

Thread diameter was formerly recorded as British Pharmacopoeia (BP) but is now usually quoted in metric gauge (Table 3.1).

KNOTS

1. A knot (strictly a bend or hitch, since a knot is a node or knob) is an intertwining of threads for the purpose of joining them. The ends of ligatures and sutures are joined in this manner. Secure fastening results from friction between threads and this is affected by the area of contact, the thread surface, the tightness of the knot and the length of thread left projecting from the knot.

Metric	0.1	0.2	0.3	0.4	0.5	0.7	1	1.5	2	3	3.5	4	5	6	7	8
Others	10/0	9/0	8/0	7/0	6/0	5/0	4/0	3/0	2/0	0	1	2	3&4	5	7	

Table 3.1 A comparison of thread sizes. At the top are the metric sizes, with the equivalent BP and BPC gauges below. Metric size numbers divided by 10 give minimal thread diameter in millimetres. 'Others' include non-absorbables and synthetic absorbables.

Key points

- As you read these accounts of knot-tying, have a length of string attached to a convenient base so you can practise the movements. This does not give you skill. It demonstrates what movements you must repeat many, many times, until you become skilled — that is, able to tie knots, without thinking, perfectly every time.
- Recognize that in all these descriptions the loose ends are kept under complete control so that you do not need to look for them. They can be passed from finger to finger or finger to instrument.

2. The half-hitch (also called an overhand hitch), forms the basis of most knots used in surgery. Cross two threads to form a closed loop (Fig. 3.2); pass one end through the loop. A half-hitch may be formed by crossing one thread over or under the other, thus making two forms of half-hitch possible (Fig. 3.3).

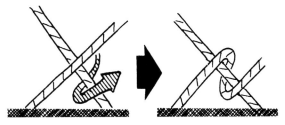

Fig. 3.2 Forming a half-hitch. Cross the threads and pass one end under the crossing to emerge on the other side.

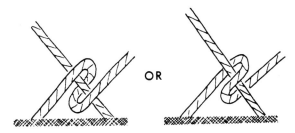

Fig. 3.3 Two types of half-hitch: starting left over right or right over left.

 Key point

- If the two ends are to be tied in a half-hitch, they must be crossed and tightened on the opposite sides of the knot from which they started (Fig. 3.4).

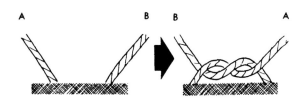

Fig. 3.4 When forming a half-hitch the ends *must* be crossed and drawn in opposite directions. Note that end A starts on the left but ends on the right, and end B starts on the right and ends on the left.

3. After tying one half-hitch, form a second half-hitch of the same type to produce a granny knot (Fig. 3.5), which has much greater holding power than a single half-hitch. Alternatively, after tying one half-hitch, form the ends into a second half-hitch of different type, producing a reef knot (the knot used when gathering a ship's sail to reef, or shorten it, Fig.3.6). In the granny knot the threads of the two half-hitches cross rather than run parallel as in the reef knot, shortening the length of contact. Note the difference, by looking down on the knots. Following the tying of a reef knot the ends lie parallel to the standing parts. Following the tying of a granny knot the ends tend to lie at right angles to the standing part (Fig. 3.7).

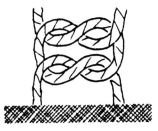

Fig. 3.5 Granny knot. Follow the path of the threads; for the first half-hitch, the left thread was passed in front of the right one, then underneath, to emerge in front on the right side. For the second half-hitch, the new left thread (the former right thread) is also passed in front of the new right thread (the former left thread) and emerges in front on the right.

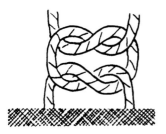

Fig. 3.6 Reef knot. The left thread was passed behind the right thread for the first half-hitch, then under it through the loop and taken to the right. The right thread emerges on the left. For the second hitch the new left thread passes in front of the new right, passes under it to emerge on the right.

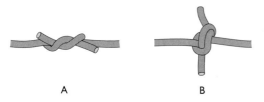

A   B

Fig. 3.7 **A** Looking down at a reef knot. The ends lie parallel to the standing threads. In **B** the ends tend to project at right angles to the standing parts – this is a granny knot.

4. If you create the same half-hitches as for a granny and a reef knot but keep one thread taut, you produce a slip knot. In the days of square-rigged ships, sailors used the reef knot not only because it was secure but because it could be easily and rapidly released. Pull one thread straight and it produces a slip knot (Fig. 3.8). The two half-hitches can be slid off the straight, standing thread. This emphasizes the critical

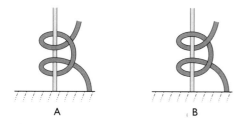

A   B

Fig. 3.8 Two varieties of slip knot. **A** The result of pulling one thread of a reef knot straight – or keeping it straight while you form it. The other thread is converted to form two half-hitches round it. **B** The result of pulling one thread of a granny knot. Note that the other thread is converted to form the well-known clove hitch round it (clove = past participle of cleave, from OE clifian = to unite, adhere).

need to tighten the knots correctly as well as forming them correctly, when you need to secure them.

5. After tying a reef knot, form a third half-hitch, making a reef knot with the second half-hitch, to produce a triple throw knot (Fig. 3.9). This is even more reliable and is used as the standard method in surgery.

6. The hands that control the ends must either cross each other or exchange ends. If they are crossed in the horizontal plane after the manner of crossing hands at the pianoforte (Fig. 3.10), they obscure the knot as they cross. If the hands pass each other in the sagittal plane, towards and away from the body (Fig. 3.11), the knot is not obscured at any time. You may be able to tie knots in the sagittal plane by adjusting your posture, either physically or mentally.

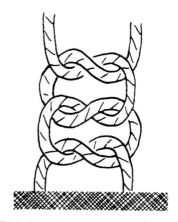

Fig. 3.9 Triple throw knot.

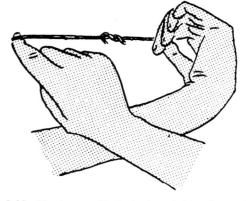

Fig. 3.10 Hands crossed in the horizontal plane obscure the field and are less in control.

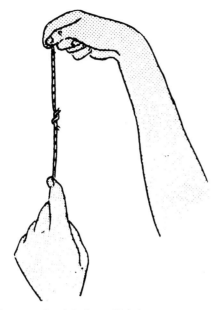

Fig. 3.11 Cross your hands in the sagittal plane.

Two-handed knot

> ### Key point
>
> - I believe this is the safest knot. Why? Both hands are actively involved and sense exactly the tension on the threads, which must be even, ensuring that you do not distort the knot or pull on their attachment. At all stages you are fully in control of the thread ends, and of the direction and amount of tension, matching them on each side.

1. If the short end of thread is towards you, pick it up between the thumb and index finger of the pronated left hand. Grip the longer end with the fully flexed right ring and little fingers, allowing the spare thread to hang from the curled little finger, leaving the thumb, index and middle fingers free. Draw a loop of the long thread to the left behind the short thread, using the left ring finger (Fig. 3.12). Pronate the right hand to thrust the right thumb under the crossing of the threads, away from you (Fig. 3.13), and trap it between the thumb and the right index finger. Release the short thread with your left hand and fully supinate your right hand (Fig. 3.14),

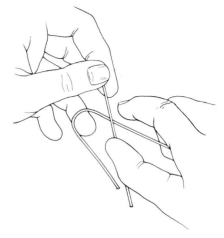

Fig. 3.12 While grasping the short thread between thumb and index finger of your pronated left hand, draw a loop of the long thread to the left, behind the vertically held short thread.

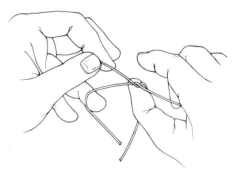

Fig. 3.13 Fully pronate your right hand in order to place your thumb under the crossing of the threads. Trap the crossing with your index finger. Now release your grasp of the short end by left thumb and index finger.

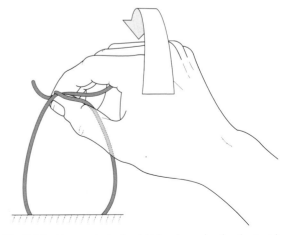

Fig. 3.14 Now supinate the right hand, carrying the short end over and back under the crossing to point towards you.

carrying the short end under the crossing of threads so that it points towards you (Fig. 3.15). Grasp the end once more between the left thumb and index finger and take it away from you as you draw the long thread in your right hand toward you, to tighten the hitch (Fig. 3.16).

2. If the short end of the thread is away from you, pick it up between the thumb and index finger of the pronated left hand. Grip the longer thread with the fully flexed ring and little fingers of the right hand, letting the spare thread hang from the curled little finger, leaving the right thumb, index and middle fingers free. Draw a loop of the long thread to the left in front of the short thread, using your left ring finger (Fig. 3.17). Supinate your right hand to thrust your index finger under the crossing of the threads, pointing towards yourself (Fig. 3.18). Release the short thread with your left hand as you trap the crossing with your right thumb (Fig. 3.19). Now fully pronate your right hand, carrying the short end under the loop to emerge on the other side, pointing away from you (Fig. 3.20). Capture the end of the short thread again with your left index finger and

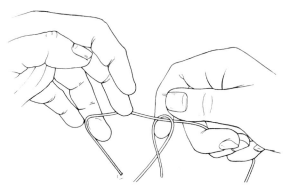

Fig. 3.15 The short end now points towards you, to be recaptured by the left hand.

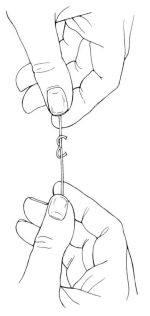

Fig. 3.16 Grasp the end of the short end between thumb and index finger of your left hand and carry it away, while drawing the long thread towards you with your right hand.

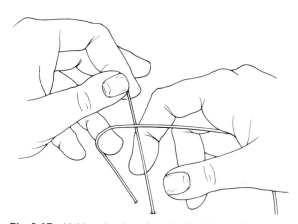

Fig. 3.17 Hold up the short thread with the index finger and thumb of your pronated left hand. Pull a loop of the long thread in front of the short thread with your left ring finger.

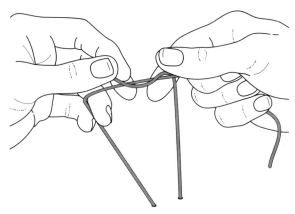

Fig. 3.18 Place the index finger of the fully supinated right hand under the crossing of the threads.

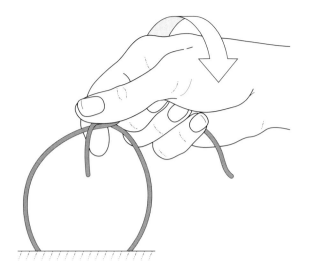

Fig. 3.19 Trap the crossing with the thumb of your fully supinated right hand as you release the short end. Fully pronate your right hand to carry the short end under the crossing, to point away from you.

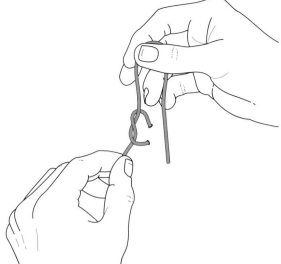

Fig. 3.21 Draw the short thread toward you and take the long thread away to tighten the half-hitch.

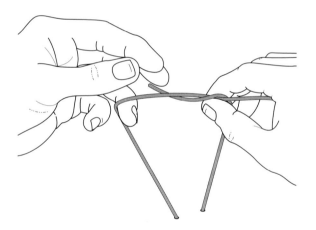

Fig. 3.20 As the short end emerges from under the crossing, pointing away from you, capture it once more with the left hand.

One-handed knot tied with the left hand

> **Key point**
>
> • I deprecate the use of this knot by trainees. It is not a bad knot but it is a badly executed knot. It looks elegant and showy – but rapidly thrown half-hitches badly laid are dangerous. Prefer slower, secure, two-handed knots unless you are confident that every hitch is not only formed but tightened perfectly every time.

thumb and draw it toward you as you take the long thread in your right hand away from you to tighten the hitch (Fig. 3.21).

3. If you start with the short end toward you, tie the hitch and carry straight on to tie the hitch with the short end pointing away from you. If you start with the short end pointing away from you, tie the hitch and carry straight on to tie the hitch with the short end pointing toward you.

1. Why tied with the left hand? If you have a free right (dominant) hand, you can tie a two-handed knot. It is the psychological immobilization of the instrument-holding hand, prejudicing the correct laying and tightening of the knot, that endangers its security.

2. A claimed advantage of this knot is that you can often hold an instrument in the right hand while forming the knot with your left hand.

3. As with the two-handed knot, there are two types of half-hitch. When the short end is away from you, use the index finger (index finger hitch). When

the short end is close to you, use the middle finger (middle finger hitch). The index finger hitch and the middle finger hitch must be tied alternately to produce a reef knot.

4. For the index-finger hitch, when the short end is away from you, pick up the short end with the thumb and middle finger of the left hand and hold it vertically. Flex the wrist so your left hand hangs from it then supinate your hand and extend the index finger to create a loop of the short thread over it. Pick up the long thread with your right hand and hold it vertically. Raise the long thread held in the right hand so that it crosses the short thread in the section between the index finger and the grasp of the middle finger and thumb of your left hand (Fig. 3.22). Flex the terminal interphalangeal joint of your left index finger round the long thread to reach behind the short thread (Fig. 3.23). The short thread lies against your nail on the dorsum of the finger. As you pronate your left hand, extend the tip of the left index finger, carrying the loop of short thread under the loop of long thread (Fig. 3.24). Release the middle finger contact with the thumb of the left hand to allow the

end of the short thread to be carried through, and use the middle finger to trap the emerging end against the index finger (Fig. 3.25). Now bring the short end toward you and take the long end away from you to tighten the hitch (Fig. 3.26).

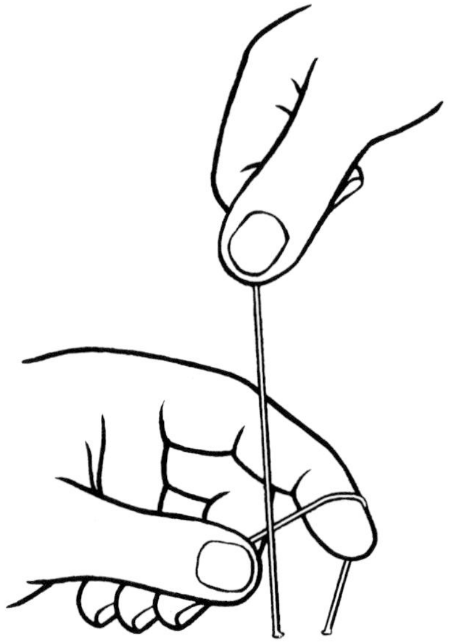

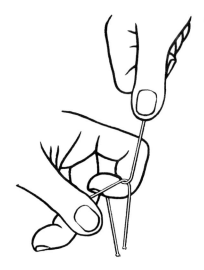

Fig. 3.23　Flex your left index finger around the vertically held long thread so that you can pull a loop of long thread up with the pulp of the index finger, while the short thread crosses the nail.

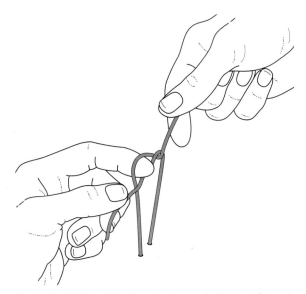

Fig. 3.22　One-handed knot with the left hand. Hold the short end between the thumb and middle finger of the pronated left hand. Supinate the left hand, swinging the left index finger to push a loop of short thread behind and beyond the long thread held vertically in the right hand. This is the index finger half-hitch.

Fig. 3.24　While still holding the short end with the left thumb and middle finger, pronate your left hand, carrying the loop of short thread under the loop of long thread on the back of your index finger.

thread over it toward yourself (Fig. 3.27), crossing the short thread. Flex the tip of your middle finger over the top of the horizontal section of the long thread and beneath the section of the short thread between the crossing of the threads and the grip of the left thumb and index finger; the nail of your middle finger lies in contact with the short thread (Fig. 3.28). As you pronate your left hand, extend your middle finger (Fig. 3.29), to carry the end of the short thread underneath the long thread, to point away from you, as you release the grip of your index finger and thumb on the tip, and extend your ring finger to trap the end against the middle finger (Fig. 3.30). Now carry the short end away from you and bring the long end toward you (Fig. 3.31) to tighten the hitch.

5. Note that when tying the index-finger hitch you need to pick up the short thread between thumb and middle finger, leaving the index finger free; when tying the middle-finger hitch you need to pick up the short thread between thumb and index finger, leaving the middle finger free.

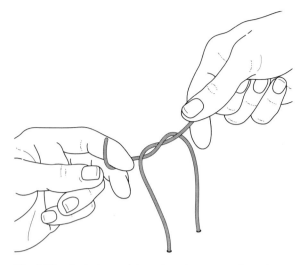

Fig. 3.25 As the loop of short thread emerges, release the left thumb and middle finger grip on the end of the short thread and use your middle finger to trap the emerging end of short thread against the index finger to be replaced by your thumb.

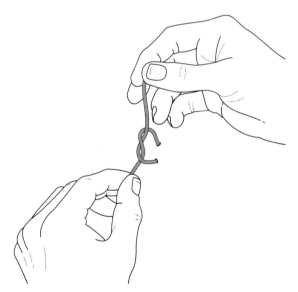

Fig. 3.26 Now draw the short end towards you and take the long end away to tighten the hitch.

4. For the middle-finger hitch, when the short end lies near you, pick it up between the index finger and thumb of the pronated left hand and hold it vertically. Pick up the long thread with your right hand and hold it vertically. Supinate your left hand as you extend the middle finger between the near short thread and the far long thread and pull the long

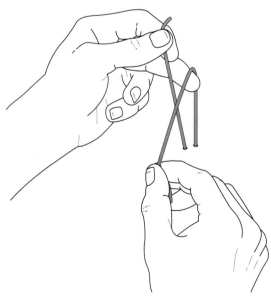

Fig. 3.27 When the short end lies near to you, pick it up between the index finger and thumb of your left hand and pick up the long thread with your right hand. Supinate your left hand and extend your middle finger, behind the short thread. Draw the long thread over the extended finger from the far side, pointing toward you. This is the middle finger half-hitch.

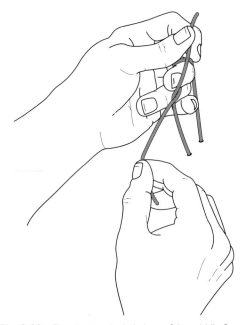

Fig. 3.28 Flex the terminal phalanx of the middle finger, to pass over the long thread but behind the part of the short thread above the crossing of the threads. The nail lies in contact with the short thread.

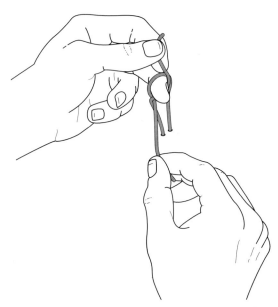

Fig. 3.29 Extend the terminal phalanx of your middle finger to carry a loop of the short thread away from you, under the long thread as you pronate your left hand..

6. An alternative to the middle-finger hitch might be called the three-finger hitch. When the short end lies near you, pick up the short end between the index finger and thumb of the pronated left hand and hold it vertically. Supinate your left hand while extending the medial three fingers so that the short thread lies on the little, ring and middle fingers. Take the long thread over the middle finger from the far side and across the ring and little fingers, coming towards you (Fig. 3.32). Flex the terminal

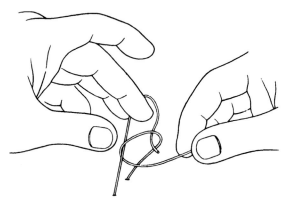

Fig. 3.30 As the loop of the short thread emerges, release the end so that it is carried through; move your left ring finger to trap the end against the middle finger.

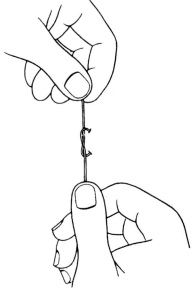

Fig. 3.31 Tighten the half-hitch by taking the short end away from you and drawing the long thread toward you.

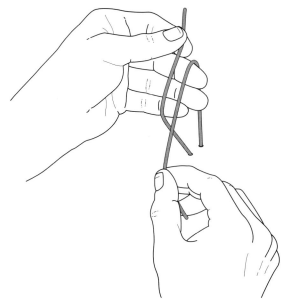

Fig. 3.32. 'Three-finger hitch'. When the short thread is closer to you, pick it up with your index finger and thumb of the pronated left hand. Now supinate your left hand but instead of extending just your middle finger, extend the medial three fingers, allowing the short thread to stretch from the little finger to the index finger and thumb. Take the long thread in the right hand on the far side of the middle finger and lay it over the three medial fingers toward you.

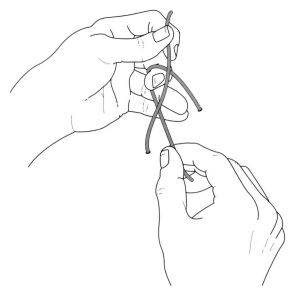

Fig. 3.33 Flex the terminal phalanx of the middle finger over the long thread and under the short thread. Prepare to extend the middle finger to draw a loop of short thread under the long thread as in Fig. 3.29.

phalanx of the left middle finger over the top of the long thread and under the section of short thread lying between the little finger and the grip of the thumb and index finger (Fig. 3.33). You can immediately trap the short thread onto the back of the middle finger, with the pulp of your ring finger. As you pronate your left hand, carry the loop of short thread under the long thread by extending the middle finger and ring fingers as in Fig. 3.29 and tighten it by taking the short thread away from you and the long thread towards you as in Fig. 3.31. The advantage of using three fingers instead of the middle finger only is that it is often easier to dip the terminal phalanx of the middle finger under the longer stretch of short thread.

Knot tied using instruments

Key point

- Use instrument ties for repetitive routine knot-tying as when inserting a line of interrupted skin stitches. Do not use the method indiscriminately. When tying important knots revert to the two-handed method.

1. The method avoids the need to put down the needle-holder to tie two-handed knots. However, instruments can be 'palmed' – held by the medial fingers while using the lateral fingers to perform manoeuvres such as knot-tying (see Ch. 2, p. 11). A less justifiable reason for using instrument ties is that the method is economical of suture material, since the short end need be only long enough to be grasped by the instrument, but this tempts you to hold it taut so the long thread forms a slip knot around it.

2. If the short end is away from you and the longer thread toward you, lay the needle-holder (it may be a haemostat or dissecting forceps – but I shall not continue to repeat this), on the long thread (Fig. 3.34). Take the long thread closest to you and pass it over the tip of the needle-holder, round it and back toward you (Fig. 3.35). While maintaining the loop, manoeuvre the needle-holder through it so you can grasp the short end (Fig.

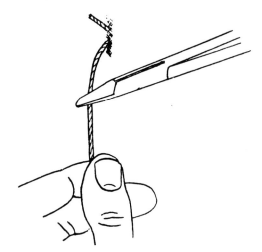

Fig. 3.34 If the short thread is farthest from you, lay the needle-holder on the long thread nearer to you.

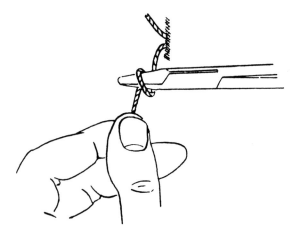

Fig. 3.35 Take a turn of thread round it.

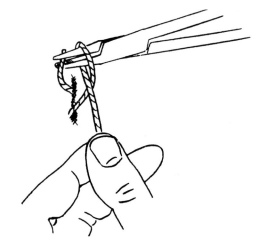

Fig. 3.36 Reach through the loop to grasp the short end.

3.36), and draw it back through the loop toward you, while taking the long thread away from you to tighten it (Fig. 3.37).

3. If the short end is near to you, take the long thread away. Lay the needle-holder on top of the long thread (Fig. 3.38). Take a turn of the thread around it (Fig. 3.39), then grasp the short end through the loop (Fig. 3.40) and draw it through. Tighten the hitch by taking the short thread away from you and drawing the long thread toward you (Fig. 3.41).

4. Knot tying using instruments only has been brought to a fine art during minimal access surgical procedures, but this is not a basic technique. Try practising the technique.

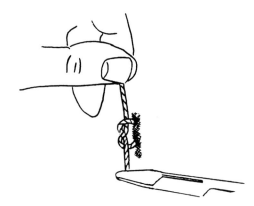

Fig. 3.37 Draw the short end through the loop towards you and take the long thread away from you to tighten the hitch.

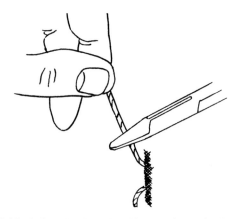

Fig. 3.38 When the short thread is towards you, lay the needle-holder on the long thread lying away from you.

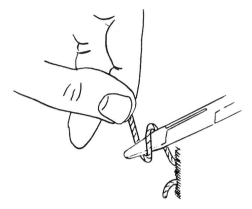

Fig. 3.39 Take a turn of the long thread around the needle-holder.

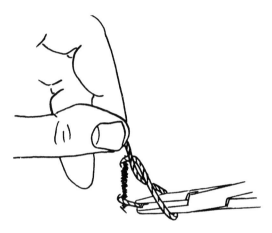

Fig. 3.40 Grasp the short end through the loop.

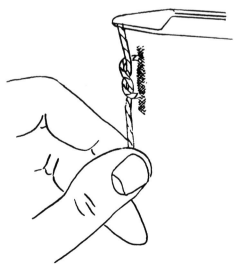

Fig. 3.41 Carry the short end through the loop and take it away from you while drawing the long thread toward you.

LAYING AND TIGHTENING KNOTS

 Key points

- Arranging the threads to lie in the correct relationship to each other is as important as forming the knots correctly.
- A carefully tightened knot weakens the thread significantly. A roughly tightened knot weakens it critically.

1. Before you tighten a hitch ensure that the loops are of equal size. We automatically move our hands apart at equal speeds. If one loop is larger than the other, the shorter one tends to become tautly straight before the slack is taken up by the other (Fig. 3.42). This fault occurs particularly when you attempt to tie a knot when one end is short. To avoid losing it, you tend to keep it taut. Once you have secured it, slacken it off until you have drawn the longer end through to match it. Plastic surgeons often pull the thread through when stitching, to leave a protruding end so short that when they have tied the knot they need to cut only the long thread. In such circumstances it is very important to lay and tighten the knot correctly.

4. The force and direction of pull for both threads must be equal and lie along a straight line passing through the centre of the knot. Any other force or

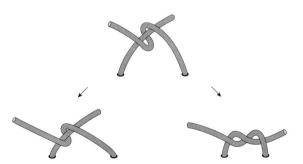

Fig. 3.42 When one end is short there is a temptation to hold it taut while tying the other thread around it. You **must** slacken the short thread while taking up the slack on the longer thread or you will produce a slipping hitch, as on the left. Only by allowing the short thread to slacken and distort will you create a true half-hitch, as on the right.

direction displaces the knot and puts traction on the attached tissues.

5. Carefully adjust the tension of the first half-hitch. To appose tissues and encourage them to unite, do not overtighten the stitch and constrict them. Remember that following a surgical procedure inflammatory oedema is inevitable; if they are already constricted, they will die or the tie will cut out. Conversely, when you are tying a vital ligature around a major blood vessel, if the tie is too slack it will be insecure. Tighten the second hitch fully on to the first. It is the binding effect of the threads of the two hitches that secures the knot.

6. When tying an important knot on to strong tissue, be willing to 'bed down' the hitches by gently and evenly tugging the ends apart two or three times (Fig. 3.43). Tighten the second hitch on to the first in a similar manner. Finally tie and securely tighten a third half-hitch, forming a reef knot with the second.

Tightening under tension

1. Of course we should not tie under tension – but we do not always have the choice.

2. If two structures must be brought together and held there with sutures or ligatures, use your assistant's hands to draw and hold them together while you tie the knots.

3. In order to create increased contact and therefore increased friction between the threads of the first half-hitch, pass the short end twice through the closed loop. When this is pulled taut, it has less tendency to slip than a normal half-hitch. Now tie a normal second half-hitch on to it to form a surgeon's knot (Fig. 3.44). I believe you should always tie a third, normal half-hitch, forming a reef knot with the second normal half-hitch. A knot in which the second hitch also has two turns is sometimes recommended – and incorrectly called a surgeon's knot. When tying smooth-surfaced, extruded synthetic material, a number of methods are recommended, such as a surgeon's knot with a third hitch having two 'throws' or turns, or a standard reef knot finished with a third hitch also having two throws (Fig. 3.45).

4. If you are tying a thread around a structure that cannot be compressed by your assistant, such as a bulky elastic duct, then the thread itself must be

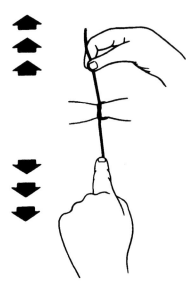

Fig. 3.43 'Bed down' the hitch on a thick structure by gently pulling the threads apart several times.

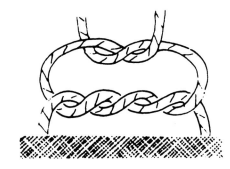

Fig. 3.44 This is a true surgeon's knot. The first half-hitch has two 'throws' or turns. The second is a standard half-hitch; I believe it should be finished off with a third half-hitch that forms a reef knot with the second half-hitch.

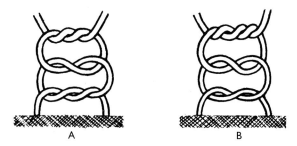

A   B

Fig. 3.45 Recommended knots for tying synthetic absorbable materials. **A** A double throw, then a single throw, followed by a double throw. **B** Tie a reef knot, then add a double throw.

capable of constricting and holding tight while you form and tighten a second hitch on to it. Try keeping the threads taut after tying and tightening the first half-hitch while you form the second hitch and tighten it onto the first (Fig. 3.46).

5. Particularly when suturing skin, the edges tend to separate after you have brought them together with the first half-hitch, which gives while you are forming and tightening the second half-hitch. Try rotating the threads clockwise or anticlockwise, to lock them (Fig. 3.47). They will lock only in one direction, depending on which type of half-hitch you have tied. As you tighten the

second hitch they unlock to form a secure reef knot but only if you form and tighten the second hitch correctly.

6. If you deliberately keep one thread taut as you throw two half-hitches around it, to form a slip knot (Fig. 3.8), you can tighten it, to be held temporarily by the friction of the threads, while you now add two correctly formed and tightened hitches to make a reef knot.

7. One of the most effective methods is to ask your assistant to compress the tightened first half-hitch with a finger while you form and tighten the second hitch, leading the tightening loop under the compressing finger (Fig. 3.48). Take care that you do not capture a small piece of the assistant's surgical glove, which will tear off when the finger is removed.

8. A valuable method is to insert one or more temporary stitches to draw separated edges together while you insert and tie the definitive stitches, and then remove them (Fig. 3.49). You may tie them, or merely cross the ends and have your assistant hold them taut.

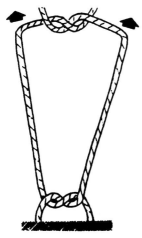

Fig. 3.46   Tying a knot under tension. After tying and tightening the first half-hitch, keep the threads taut while you form and tighten the second hitch, to stop the first hitch from slipping.

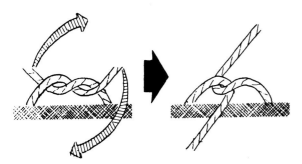

Fig. 3.47   After tying and tightening the first half-hitch, rotate the ends clockwise or anticlockwise to 'lock' the threads while you tie and tighten the second hitch onto it. You must rotate the threads correctly and you **must** tie and tighten the second hitch correctly to create a reef knot.

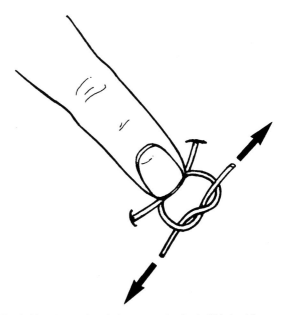

Fig. 3.48   Your assistant's finger traps the first half-hitch while you tie the second half-hitch. You must lead the tightening threads under the assistant's finger – without capturing part of the glove.

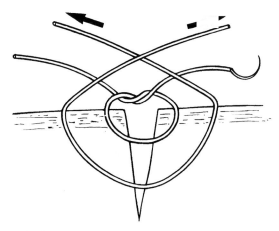

Fig. 3.49 Insert and tie a temporary stitch to take the tension while you insert and tie the definitive stitches. You need not tie it if you have your assistant cross the threads and hold them taut.

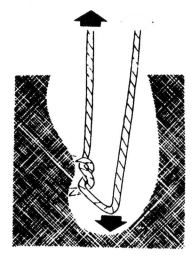

Fig. 3.51 When tightening a knot within a cavity, you must push one end in with exactly the force with which you pull the other end out. If not, you will displace the structure, or pull off the ligature.

Tying knots in cavities

1. In some cases you need to tie a knot deep in a cavity. As a rule it is most convenient to form the hitches outside the cavity.

2. Ensure that you have a sufficient length of thread so that after you have encircled or sutured the deep structure both ends of the thread lie outside the cavity.

3. Tie a two-handed half-hitch outside the cavity (Fig. 3.50) without putting any tension on the threads.

4. With an extended finger, or a pushed but not grasping instrument, close the loop on to the structure.

5. Tighten the hitch by pushing down with a finger on one thread, with exactly the same force as you pull on the other thread from outside the cavity (Fig. 3.51).

In some cases, when you can insert both hands, you can pull the threads apart as you would on the surface.

> **Key point**
>
> - If you merely pull on the deep structure you may damage it, or pull off the tie.

LIGATURES

1. A ligature (L *ligare* = to bind) is tied round a structure, most commonly a blood vessel or other duct, and is usually intended to close the lumen. Ligatures are secured by knotting the ends. Blood-vessel ligation is one of the commonest repetitive procedures in surgery.

> **Key point**
>
> - Practise, practise, practise ligating vessels until you can perform it effortlessly, perfectly, every time. Perfection is more important than time. Indeed, two rapidly performed failed attempts take longer than a single effective ligature.

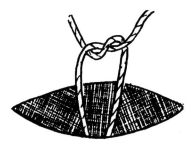

Fig. 3.50 Tying a knot in a cavity. Form the hitches on the surface, so ensure the thread is sufficiently long.

2. Silk, linen and cotton are soft, flexible, can be tied securely without slipping and have a limited tendency to be reabsorbed. Avoid using them near the skin unless you will remove them, because the foreign body reaction they generate may produce worrying subcutaneous nodules or even sinuses to the skin surface.

3. Synthetic polymerised absorbable threads are digested with minimum inflammation, usually by hydrolysis. Springy stainless steel and synthetic non-absorbable material cause minimal tissue reaction but are usually now restricted to binding together solid structures such as bone.

4. Select the finest material that will reliably hold. Position it, tie and tighten it carefully. Too tight a ligature cuts through fragile tissue, too slack and it will not occlude a thick-walled vessel or it will slip off.

5. When preparing to divide and ligate ducts and blood vessels, preferably doubly clamp and divide them first or clamp them after they are cut. In either circumstance place the forceps with the concavity towards the cut and ensure that the tips of the forceps project a few millimetres beyond the ducts or vessels.

6. While an assistant holds up the handles of the haemostatic forceps, pass the end of the ligature under them on the side away from you, to capture it with the other hand (Fig. 3.52). Alternatively,

stretch the thread between your hands on the far side of the forceps and then have your assistant reach over the thread and pick up the handles (Fig. 3.53)

7. When passing ligatures round vessels or ducts placed deeply, carry the thread stretched between the tips of your index fingers (Fig. 3.54) in order to reach under the tips of the forceps to avoid incorporating them in the ligature. Alternatively, use dissecting or artery forceps (Fig. 3.55) or an aneurysm needle. Warn your assistant to avoid pulling on the forceps; they will be pulled off or allow the ligature to slip over the tips of the forceps. Avoid tying in the tips of the forceps or, when they are removed, the ligature will be pulled off.

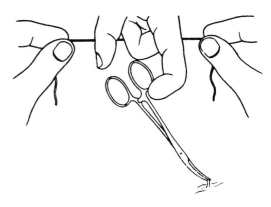

Fig. 3.53 Stretch the thread between your hands beyond the forceps and have your assistant reach over the thread to pick up the handle of the forceps.

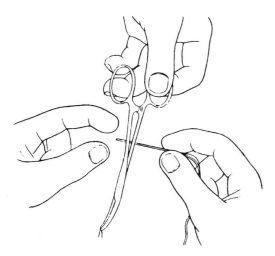

Fig. 3.52 While your assistant lifts the handles of the forceps, pass the ligature from one hand to the other behind them.

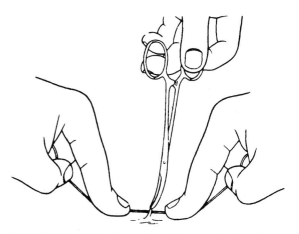

Fig. 3.54 Stretch the ligature thread between the tips of your index fingers to depress it and encircle only the vessel, without including the tips of the forceps.

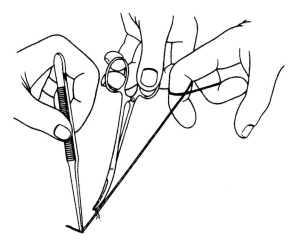

Fig. 3.55 You may pass the ligature using long-handled dissecting forceps.

8. Tie the ligature carefully, slowly and securely.

9. Do not let your assistant undo all your safety precautions by cutting the threads too short. Have the ends of silk, linen or braided materials cut 2–3 mm long, and monofilamentous materials cut to 4–5 mm.

STITCHES

1. Versatile thread stitches are peerless for joining together tissues that can be pierced with a needle, in spite of the development of metal clips and adhesives. Threads are carried through by the needle and secured by knotting them.

2. Suture strength is related to the diameter of any particular material and is measured by 'knot pull strength' test – the force that can be applied to the free ends of a suture tied with a surgical knot around a quarter-inch rubber tube.

3. A portion of tissue may need to be constricted to stop or prevent bleeding or leakage of internal fluids.

4. To prevent a ligature around a divided duct or vessel from slipping, first insert a stitch across the diameter of the tube, then tie it as a suture–ligature.

5. A stitch left long and untied can act as a means of exerting gentle traction.

6. A coloured-thread stitch makes a convenient marker.

7. If two materials are to be joined, insert the stitch through one, then the other, and knot the ends of the threads together.

8. A weak area can be reinforced by inserting a darn (Fig. 3.56). Run the stitch back and forth without being pulled tight. The strands are interwoven in fabric darns but this cannot always be carried out in surgical practice.

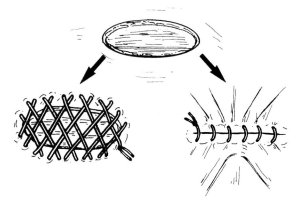

Fig. 3.56 Closing a defect. Instead of dragging the edges together under tension, as on the right, bridge it with a darn. Ideally, the darn threads interlock in the manner of woven fabric, although this is not always carried out.

NEEDLES

1. Needles come in a variety of shapes and sizes (Fig. 3.57). Curved needles are most commonly used. As a general rule they follow the circumference of a circle and may be only a small arc or more than half the circumference.

2. Straight, hand-held needles were formerly used extensively in surgery (Fig. 3.58). Surgeons are expert in handling them – flexible structures can be deformed in order to facilitate the entrance and exit of a straight needle to provide a curved passage of threads. The needles are so convenient that glove and skin punctures were accepted as a small price to pay. Recognition of the transmission of viral infections has made us change over exclusively to no-touch techniques. Whenever you need to use a straight needle, control it using a needle-holder (Fig. 3.59).

3. Virtually all needles are now eyeless and factory prepared. The needle is usually swaged on to the thread, although fine threads may be inserted

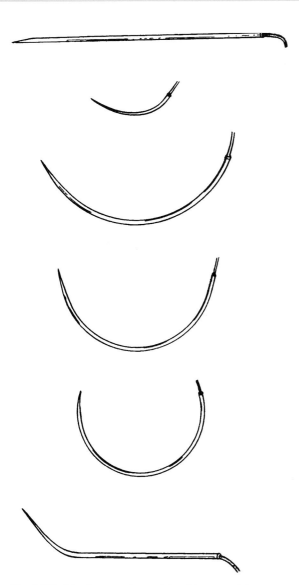

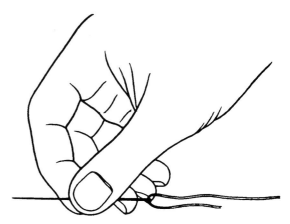

Fig. 3.58 The hand-held straight needle is convenient – but dangerous.

Fig. 3.57 Needles come in a variety of shapes and sizes.

and fixed with an adhesive into holes drilled into the shank of the needles. As a result, the hole produced by the needle is only slightly larger than the thread that will be drawn through it.

4. Sutures are supplied in sealed packets after gamma-ray sterilization.

5. A variety of points and cross-sections are available (Fig. 3.60) and the sizes range down to 3 mm for microsurgery. The needle shank is usually flattened along the section that will be grasped by the needle-holder.

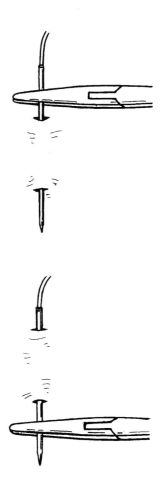

Fig. 3.59 Insert and withdraw a straight needle using a needle-holder.

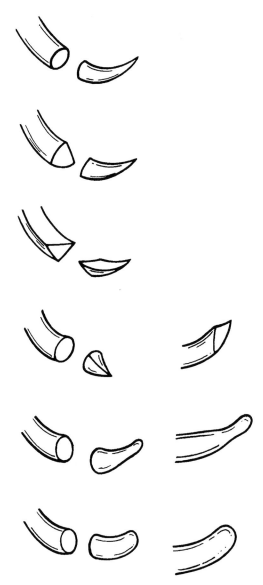

7. Skin and fibrous tissue are resistant, so use cutting needles of triangular or flat cross-section. The sharp edges of the needle cut through the tissues, so they do not contract on to the thread. Cutting needles of triangular section usually have the apex of the triangle on the inside of the curve. When such needles are used to insert stitches that will come under tension, in pulling two edges together, the threads tend to extend the split towards the edges with a liability to cut out. Reverse cutting needles have a flat surface on the inside of the curve and are less likely to cut out (Fig. 3.61). An alternative is a spear point, which is flat on the inside and outside of the curve.

8. Use blunt, taper-pointed needles for stitching soft tissues such as the abdominal wall, excluding the skin. The needles penetrate the fascia and muscles but surgical gloves usually resist penetration and so protect you from needle-stick injury.

9. Use blunt-ended, round-bodied needles to sew soft viscera such as liver. Sharp-edged needles create splits that are likely to extend.

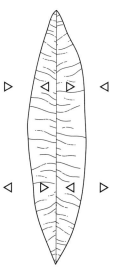

Fig. 3.60 Needle cross-sections and points. From above downwards: round-bodied taper-point, triangular cutting, reversed cutting, trocar pointed, blunt taper point, and blunt-ended.

6. Use a round-bodied needle to sew fragile tissue or tissue arranged in strands that can be displaced, since the strands are not cut, merely pushed aside, with minimal damage. Round-bodied needles are appropriate for sewing bowel and blood vessels because the round holes produced by the passage of the needle close by tissue elasticity around the thread, preventing leakage.

Fig. 3.61 Closing a wound that is under tension or is liable to be put under tension. Top: the holes made by a standard cutting needle with the apex of the triangle on the inside of the curve. It is liable to extend when subjected to tension. Bottom: the holes made by a reversed cutting needle present a flat face to the site of possible tension when the suture is tied. There is less likelihood of such a suture cutting out if it is placed under tension.

10. Use a robust trocar (F *trois* = three + *carré* = side) needle when sewing very tough tissues in which a normal needle might break.

> ### 🔑 Key points
>
> - Do not pick up needles with your fingers. Use needle-holders and forceps to control them. Never leave them where they could damage your patient, yourself or your colleagues.
> - When not in use, place them in a kidney dish. Never pass them from hand to hand.
> - Many needle pricks occur during abdominal wall closure; the blunt taper-point needle effectively penetrates the tissues of the abdominal wall but glove penetration is greatly reduced.

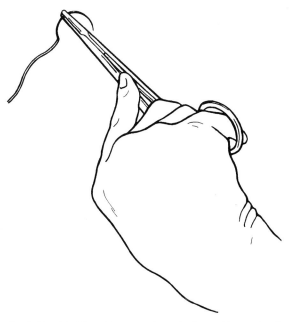

Fig. 3.62 Stitching with a curved needle. Start with your hand fully pronated.

Stitching with a curved needle

1. Insert and withdraw curved needles exclusively with instruments. The tissues can usually be moulded to conform to the curvature.

2. Do not select too short a needle. You need to have sufficient length to allow you to push in the needle and retain a grip until the point emerges sufficiently to be gripped without damaging the point. For the same reason, do not attempt to take large bites of tissue on each side of a suture line in a single pass. Prefer to take the needle through each side separately.

3. Mount the needle in the tip of the needle-holder, approximately one-third of the way from the threaded end towards the point. If you are right-handed, with your hand in mid-pronation, the needle-holder pointing away from you, have the needle point upwards and to the left, upwards and to the right if you stitch with your left hand. Right-handed operators most easily stitch from right to left, and from away towards you. Left-handed operators prefer to stitch from left to right, and from away towards you.

4. Start with the hand fully pronated to enter the tissues perpendicularly (Fig. 3.62, see also Fig. 3.65A). As you continue, progressively supinate the hand so that the path follows the curve of the needle (Fig. 3.63). In this way the needle finally emerges perpendicularly from the tissues (Fig. 3.64).

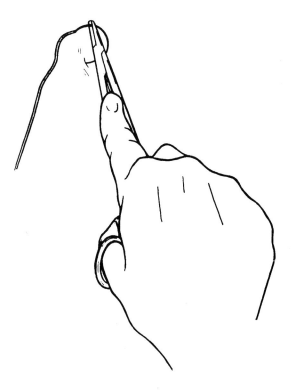

Fig. 3.63 Needle driven in a curved path by progressively supinating your hand.

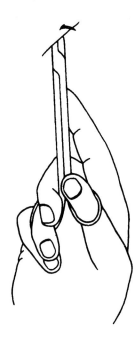

Fig. 3.64 Your wrist is fully supinated as the needle emerges.

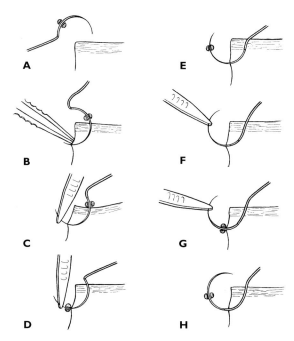

Fig. 3.65 Diagram illustrating the insertion of a stitch using a curved needle held in a needle-holder, indicated by two apposed stippled hemispheres. It shows a right-handed surgeon inserting the stitch from dominant to non-dominant side. If you are left-handed the needle is inserted in the opposite direction. **A** Enter the point at right angles to the surface; your hand is fully pronated. **B** As you drive the needle through, progressively supinating your hand, apply counterpressure against the tissues as the point emerges, so helping to reveal more of the needle. **C** When sufficient needle emerges, grasp and steady it with dissecting forceps. **D** Release the needle-holder and re-apply it to the emerging needle. **E** Draw through the needle along its curved path. **F** Steady the needle with the dissecting forceps. **G** Re-apply the needle-holder to the emerging needle at the place you wish to grasp it for the next stitch, keeping your hand partly supinated. **H** Finally, draw the needle right through, with a fully supinated hand.

 Key point

- The ability to pronate and supinate enables you to drive a curved needle through the tissues with minimal trauma, and with minimal force. Make full use of this human facility. The range of movement can be extended by shoulder and trunk movements.

5. If necessary, use the closed tips of dissecting forceps to apply counterpressure near, but not on, the point of emergence of the needle in order to avoid turning the needle point and blunting it (Fig. 3.65B). If you use too short a needle, or take too great a bite, you may need to change the grasp of the needle-holder nearer the thread end of the needle, in order to push the needle further through. When the point comes into view, grasp the shank behind it, if necessary gently pushing back the surface tissue to expose a greater length of needle, and steady it (Fig. 3.65C).

6. Relinquish the grasp of the needle-holder and use it to re-grasp the emerging needle, gently pushing back the tissues to allow you to grasp it well away from the point (Fig. 3.65D).

7. Draw the needle through along its curved path (Fig. 3.65E) by further supinating your hand.

8. Again steady the needle with the dissecting forceps so you can disengage the needle-holder (Fig. 3.65F).

9. Re-grasp the needle in the correct position for making the next stitch (Fig. 3.65G), and draw it through (Fig. 3.65H). If you are inserting a continuous suture you do not need to adjust the needle-holder.

> ## Key point
>
> - If you select the needle size correctly to match the tissue thickness and stitch depth and length, you can avoid several steps. In one movement you may expose enough emerging needle to be able to grasp it far enough back so that you can replace the needle-holder in the correct position for the next stitch. However, if you pronate your hand before grasping the emerging needle, you will need to change your grip before inserting the next stitch. Try it.

10. When stitching in difficult circumstances you may need to stitch from non-dominant to dominant-hand direction, or from near to far. Sometimes you can avoid this by going to the other side of the operating table. If not, take especial care. You will be made aware of the difference in facility between making a familiar and an unfamiliar manoeuvre.

11. Do not draw through the thread by pulling on the needle. You risk sticking the needle into an assistant or pulling the needle off the thread. Grasp the thread with a spare finger of the hand holding the needle-holder. Above all, do not draw through the thread by grasping it with the needle-holder or dissecting forceps; all the modern threads are severely weakened by being held with metal instruments.

12. Watch spare thread as you stitch. It has a fiendish propensity to catch on any projections. Have your assistant follow it and guide it; if you are using stainless steel you must avoid producing kinks. Do not try to stitch with thread of too short a length – you are tempted to take shorter stitches, tie imperfect knots and waste time.

TYPES OF STITCH (FIG. 3.66)

> ## Key point
>
> - Surgeons often adamantly claim that the type of stitch they use is the reason for their success. They are too modest (a characteristic rarely attributed to surgeons). Their success depends on the care with which they stitch. Watch a few outstanding surgeons performing – the only common factor is the perfection of their technique, not the methods they use

1. The simplest stitch to join two edges of tissue is a single thread that catches each side and draws them into contact, with both ends of the thread tied with a reef knot. This is an *interrupted stitch*. Pierce the tissue perpendicular to the upper and lower surfaces, otherwise it has an inverting or everting effect. If you tie it too tightly, or if it is subjected to too much tension, either the thread will break or it will cut out.

2. A *mattress stitch* is a double stitch. Start from one side, cross to the other side, re-insert the needle at a small distance from where it emerged and take it through to emerge on the original side a short

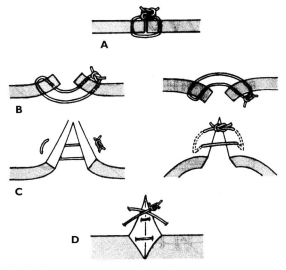

Fig. 3.66 Commonly used stitches. **A** Simple interrupted. **B** Interrupted longitudinal mattress, everting on the left, inverting on the right. **C** Interrupted horizontal mattress, everting on the left, inverting on the right. **D** Inverting 'X' stitch.

distance from the first entry and tie the original entry and final exit thread together. Because a mattress stitch draws on a segment of tissue between the two lengths of thread joining the edges, it is much less likely to cut out. This is particularly true when you sew tissues in which the fibres run at right angles to the edges (Fig. 7.6, p. 119).

3. If the entry and exit holes lie parallel to the edges, this is a horizontal mattress stitch. If the entry and exit holes are perpendicular to the edges, one bite is smaller than the other, this is a vertical or longitudinal mattress stitch. In each case, there is a bridge of suture on the upper surface which draws in the surface away from the edge so that the edge itself is everted. These are therefore referred to as *everting mattress stitches*. Skin sometimes tends to invert and if you allow it to do so when closing a suture line, you are apposing the dead keratinised surface cells, so healing is delayed and imperfect, and the scar will be weak. When suturing blood vessels you must appose the endothelium, by slightly everting the edges, or clots will form on the internal suture line. As a rule you can easily get the edges to turn out using simple sutures but on occasion you may need to start the necessary eversion with one or two everting stitches.

4. In contrast, bowel should not normally be everted. The French surgeon Antoine Lembert (1802–1851) recognized that if the outer, serous coats of bowel were brought into contact, they rapidly sealed together and prevented leakage. He described in 1826 a separate row of stitches that picked up only the serous and muscular coats, placed outside the main stitches, to create an inverting effect. However, the effect can be achieved with a single row of stitches and Lembert's stitch is less frequently used than formerly. Insert an *inverting mattress stitch* by passing the suture through the wall from outside in, to the mucosal surface, returning it to the surface on the same side a short distance from the entry stitch. Now cross to the opposite side and pass the suture from outside in to the mucosal surface, returning it to the exterior from the inside out, to emerge close to the entry stitch. Tie this thread to the end of thread at the original site. You have created a mattress stitch with the loop not on the surface of the bowel but on the mucosal aspect. When the stitch is tied it tends to bring the outer, serosal surfaces together. This stitch is often named after Gregory Connell, the American surgeon who described it in 1864.

Interrupted stitches

1. These have the advantage that, when used in series, failure of one does not necessarily prejudice the other stitches.

2. The potential weakness of interrupted stitches is that each one is held by a knot; even when knots are perfectly tied and tightened they reduce the strength of the thread considerably. A roughly tied, snatched or imperfectly tightened knot may reduce the strength by over 50%. Once one knot gives way, the contiguous stitches are subjected to greater tension and may give way in turn. It is for this reason that you must form and tighten every knot perfectly, every time.

3. Moreover, tension on the stitches must be even; if they are not, the tightest stitch is exposed to excess tension and may give way, creating a domino effect. Moreover, the overtightened stitch tends to strangle the enclosed tissue and subsequently cut out.

Continuous stitches

1. These have the advantage of being quick to insert and have knots only at the beginning and the end – but **those two knots are crucial**.

2. Stitching can be carried out in a continuous manner, forming a spiral within the tissues. It has the advantage that the tissues are not strangulated, although the tension is usually sufficient to be haemostatic (Fig. 3.67A).

3. You may use a variety of stitches depending on the circumstances. If you pass the needle through the loop of the previous stitch before it is tightened, you produce a locked stitch, which holds the tension while the next stitch is inserted (Fig. 3.67B) – but do not drag the thread through the loop or you will damage it. A continuous mattress stitch with the loops on the surface has an everting effect (Fig. 3.67C). In contrast, a stitch leaving loops on the deep surface has an inverting effect (Fig. 3.67D). In some circumstances it is an advantage to bury the stitches beneath the surface. This is especially valuable, especially when you are sewing skin, in

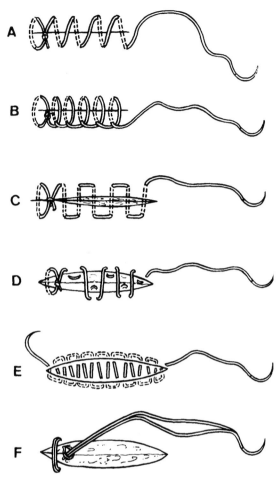

Fig. 3.67 Continuous stitches. **A** Over-and-over, spiral. **B** Locking or blanket stitch. **C** Continuous everting mattress stitch. **D** Continuous inverting mattress stitch. **E** Subcuticular type of stitch. **F** Starting a continuous run using a doubled looped thread.

anchoring the thread with the minimum bulk. Continue the stitch and, if there is sufficient length at the point of closure, cut one thread near the needle, take another stitch with the remaining thread and then tie the two threads to form a knot that is not excessively bulky.

4. When inserting continuous stitches, make sure they lie correctly; guide them by holding the loop with a finger or a closed dissecting forceps (Fig. 3.68) and carefully place the thread as you tighten it.

5. Continuous stitches cause twisting of the thread. From time to time run your finger and thumb along the thread from where it emerges from the last stitch to the needle to allow the twists to unwind.

6. The union may be edge to edge, inverted or everted, controlled by the way in which you form and tighten the threads and place the edges (Fig. 3.69). When sewing bowel, if you hold back each tightening loop while pushing in the edges with a finger tip or dissecting forceps, the loop will retain an inverting effect, especially if you tighten the thread only when you have inserted the stitch from without in and you are drawing the thread from within the lumen. This is because the tightening outer loop inverts the edges. When sewing skin or blood vessels, if you evert the edges between finger and thumb or dissecting forceps, the tightening

which case it is called a subcutaneous stitch (Fig. 3.67E). I shall deal with this in more detail in Chapter 6. When inserting stitches that will be buried in tough tissue potentially subject to tension, the required strength may demand a very thick, stiff suture that is not only difficult to knot but would produce a large mass of foreign material. By using doubled thread, the thickness can be reduced and the suppleness increased. Needles can be supplied with both ends of a thread swaged into the needle, leaving a loop at the free end. Make the initial stitch and pass the needle through the loop (Fig. 3.67 F) so

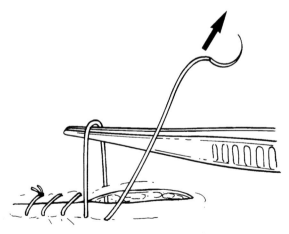

Fig. 3.68 Control the thread loop with your fingers or dissecting forceps as you tighten it, to guard against it snagging or catching on other structures and to ensure that it sits perfectly.

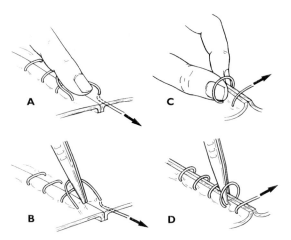

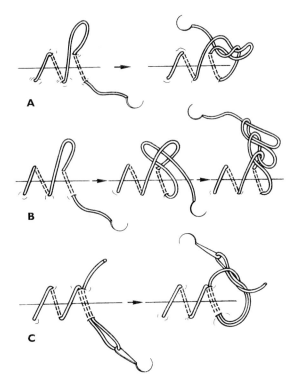

Fig. 3.69 Producing inversion and eversion using simple 'over-and-over' stitches. **A** Push in the edges and hold back the loop with your index finger as you draw the loop tight from the under surface, along the line of stitching. **B** Alternatively, achieve the same effect by the 'no touch' method, using dissecting forceps. **C** Evert the skin edges using your finger and thumb. **D** Alternatively, achieve the same effect by gently pinching the edges to maintain the eversion.

stitch will retain an everting effect. Once started, the effect of edge-to-edge, inversion or eversion tends to continue as you insert further stitches.

7. At the beginning of the run, insert the first stitch and tie it as though this is an interrupted stitch, but do not cut the thread. Continue to the end. You now have two choices to tie off this single thread. The traditional method is to hold the last loop before inserting the final stitch, using the closed loop as though it is a single thread. Having inserted the last stitch, cut off the needle and tie a knot using the final thread and the closed loop; be careful and use several throws, since knots are not as secure using threads of different thickness as when they are the same thickness (Fig. 3.70). An alternative method is to hold the loop before the last stitch, then pull a loop of the thread following the last stitch through the first loop, tighten the first loop, pass a loop of the final thread through the second loop and finally pass the needled end through that loop and tighten it. This method is used by knitters finishing off a row of knitting and by fisherman when they are repairing their nets – in honour of the fishermen of Aberdeen it is usually

Fig. 3.70 Different methods of tying off continuous sutures. **A** Hold a loop before inserting the last stitch; use this loop like a single thread to tie to the end, after cutting off the needle – I have left it on in the drawing to identify it. **B** Hold a loop before inserting the final stitch. When you have inserted the stitch, pass a loop of the free thread through the first loop, tighten the first loop, pass a third loop through the second loop and tighten the second loop and so on three or four times. Finally, pass the needle and the free end through the last loop, tighten the loops and cut off the needle, leaving a generous free end. This is often called the Aberdeen, crochet, or daisy chain knot. **C** When using an eyed needle, hold on to the free end before inserting the last stitch, and tie this to the doubled end attached to the needle. Because the threads are of unequal thickness, tie several half-hitches and securely bed them down. Finally, cut off the needle.

called an Aberdeen knot. If you happen to be using an eyed needle, you can hold on to the end of the thread before inserting the last stitch and tying this to the loop after making the stitch.

8. If you do not have sufficient thread to complete a continuous line of sutures, tie off and start again. You may leave the end of the first thread loose, insert a new stitch and tie it, then tie the loose end of the first thread to the new one.

4

Handling ducts and cavities

with Brian Davidson

The body has a variety of ducts (L *ducere* = to lead or conduct). In addition there are many closed spaces or potential spaces. Be careful to avoid inadvertent injury to normal function.

- Some ducts, such as the ureter, oesophagus and intestine, are capable of peristalsis. The circular smooth muscle contracts to occlude the lumen above, and relaxes below, the content. An intra-muscular neural plexus generates a wave of contraction preceded by relaxation, carrying the content with it. Consider the effects of any procedure on the resulting function.
- Other ducts, such as the common bile duct, have insufficient muscle to produce peristalsis; transmission of the content is by vis a tergo (L = force from behind).
- Passage of content is controlled by circular muscle sphincters, for example at the pylorus (G *pyle* = a gate + *ouros* = a watcher) and at the lower end of the bile duct – the sphincter of Oddi.
- Substances are absorbed from, and secreted or excreted into, the lumen of glands and some ducts such as the intestine.
- Passages and cavities are created by disease – sinuses and fistulas, or spaces such as seromas, haematomas, cysts and abscesses.
- Potential spaces are opened up surgically.
- Artificial fistulas include internal fistulas such as gastroenterostomy and external stomas.
- Wherever there is stagnation in spaces or in ducts, microorganisms collect and tend to contaminate and infect the tissues.

> **Key points**
>
> - Although tubes within the body differ in form and function, they are all transmitters of substances.
> - Many of them are prone to injury, stenosis, obstruction and other mechanical problems and may require intubation, dilatation, drainage, repair and anastomosis. Some cavities require similar management.

> ## Key points
>
> - The principles of management are often common to different situations. For this reason, acquire as wide a familiarity with all the techniques, watch experts and assiduously practise the manoeuvres to acquire the necessary skills. Success often results from adapting methods from one area to another.
> - I have used procedures that are life-saving or commonly performed as specific examples to demonstrate the required technical skills but have excluded selection, preparation and aftercare.
> - Blood vessels have unique characteristics that justify treating them separately.

INTUBATION

PERCUTANEOUS INTUBATION

A number of commonly performed procedures, some of them life-saving, incorporate percutaneous puncture.

1. Insert needles in a straight line; if you need to change direction it is usually best to withdraw the needle and reinsert it. If you move the needle within the tissues you may damage any or all of the structures between the entry point and the tip.

2. Hollow needles are available in varying diameters and lengths, for example long, thin, 'skinny' needles are used for percutaneous liver puncture to minimize subsequent leakage. Needles are usually best connected to a syringe so that you can see what emerges, or aspirate contents. Do not use short needles that must be fully inserted since, if they break off at the Luer connection, the thin shaft is difficult to identify and grasp.

3. When you intend to remove fluid, interpose a three-way tap between the needle and the syringe; aspirated fluid can then be expelled through the side channel of the tap into a receiver.

4. Some needles have an obturator (L *obturare* = to stop up) that is withdrawn when the needle is correctly placed, allowing contents to emerge; lumbar puncture needles have obturators, presumably to prevent the contamination of cerebrospinal fluid by other fluids during the passage of the needle.

5. If you wish to inject fluid into a tube or space, can you confirm that the tip of the needle is correctly sited? You may aspirate fluid that you can identify, such as bile when performing percutaneous trans-hepatic biliary puncture, and inject radio-opaque material to outline the biliary tract radiographically (Fig. 4.1A). You may aspirate fluid from a cyst, blood from a haematoma or pus from an abscess cavity (Fig. 4.1B). In some cases, ease of fluid injection helps confirm that the tip is in the correct place; for example, insufflation of the peritoneal cavity with carbon dioxide to initiate pneumoperitoneum does not produce a rapid rise in pressure as would occur if the gas is infused into a closed space. In contrast, when you wish to inject into a closed space such as an obstructed tube, carefully note if the flow is freer than you expect.

6. When you have entered the tube or space, make

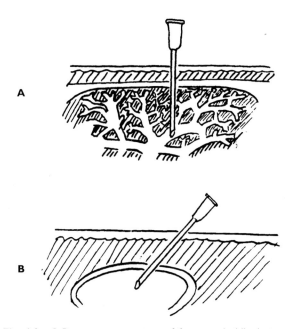

Fig. 4.1 **A** Percutaneous puncture of, for example, bile ducts within the liver. **B** Puncture of a cavity such as a cyst, haematoma or abscess cavity.

sure you do not penetrate beyond it. One method is to mark the penetrator with a clamp or the fingers, or use a penetrator with a shoulder, such as on a haemorrhoid injection needle, to limit its entrance. A similar risk occurs when creating a pneumoperi-toneum prior to minimal access surgery (see Ch. 13). To minimize the risk of penetrating the viscera within the potential space before they fall away from the parietal peritoneum (Fig. 4.2), use the special Veress needle, which has a sharp bevel tip but within it a spring-loaded blunt trocar. As soon as the bevel penetrates the parietal peritoneum the trocar projects, pushing away any at-risk viscera. In other circumstances you may not know the required depth of penetration; when entering the trachea, too deep intrusion may damage the thin posterior wall or even breach the oesophagus. Too deep insertion of the needle may cause damage during lumbar puncture or pericardiocentesis.

Cricothyroid puncture

Cricothyroid puncture may be life-saving in the absence of any other means of relieving respiratory obstruction.

1. Feel for the laryngeal prominence, follow down the anterior edge of the thyroid cartilage to the gap between the thyroid and cricoid cartilages.

2. Insert a needle carrying an external cannula, in the midline just above the cricoid cartilage, aiming slightly caudally, while aspirating on an attached syringe. Feel for the 'give' as you pierce the cricothyroid membrane. As soon as air enters the syringe you are in the trachea.

3. Hold the needle still while gently advancing the cannula. If you do not have a cannulated needle, use one or more plain needles to create an emergency short term relief.

Cricothyrotomy

Cricothyrotomy is the preferred emergency procedure.

1. Carry it out if necessary without preliminary local anaesthesia and tracheal intubation.

2. Place the patient supine, head straight, in line with the body. If possible extend the neck by placing a pillow under the upper thoracic spine.

3. Ensure that the trachea is central. Identify the thyroid cartilage. Follow the anterior border down to the gap from here to the cricoid cartilage.

4. Incise the skin transversely for 1–1.5 cm over the centre of the cricothyroid membrane and deepen it down to and through the membrane, signalled by a hiss of air (Fig. 4.3).

> **Key point**
>
> • Do not extend the incision too far laterally or you may cause bleeding from the anterior jugular veins. Avoid inserting the knife too deeply or you may penetrate the thin posterior wall into the pharynx.

Fig. 4.2 Methods of limiting overpenetration and inadvertent damage to susceptible structures. **A** Place a non-damaging clip on the puncturing instrument. **B** Use a shouldered needle, as is used for injection of haemorrhoids. **C** Grasp the instrument at a point that limits insertion. **D** The Veress needle has a blunt, spring-loaded obturator that projects as soon as resistance is overcome, pushing away at-risk mobile structures.

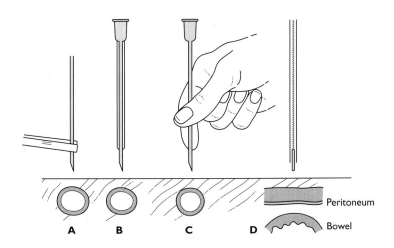

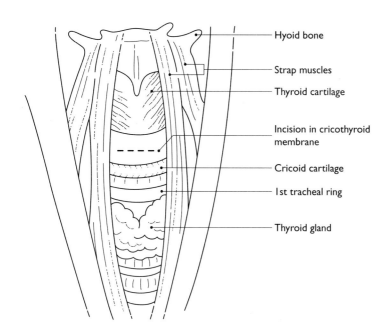

- Hyoid bone
- Strap muscles
- Thyroid cartilage
- Incision in cricothyroid membrane
- Cricoid cartilage
- 1st tracheal ring
- Thyroid gland

Fig. 4.3 Cricothyrotomy. The incision is shown in the broken line.

5. It is traditional to reverse the knife, insert the handle into the laryngeal incision and turn it to open the incision. Prefer to hold the knife blade quite still and insert alongside it a haemostatic or other forceps. Now withdraw the knife blade, open the forceps to create a gap and insert the tube alongside it.

6. Remove the forceps. If the tube has an inflatable cuff, gently expand it. If it has attached tapes, encircle the neck and tie them to secure the tube.

 Key point

- In an emergency use your ingenuity. Many lives have been saved by using penknives to insert a variety of tubes. Tracheostomy is inappropriate as an emergency procedure except when carried out by an expert.

Lumbar puncture

Lumbar puncture is usually performed with the patient lying on the side, with fully flexed spine to widen the space between the posterior vertebral arches, and the spine strictly horizontal and parallel to the couch.

1. Under strict sterile precautions, following an injection of local anaesthetic, insert the spinal needle with the lumen filled by an obturator, between the 3rd and 4th, or 4th and 5th vertebral spines, perpendicular to the skin surface or minimally angled in a cephalic direction.

2. Feel for the 'give' as you pierce the interlaminar ligament (ligamentum flavum), the depth for extradural – 'epidural' – puncture.

3. If you need to enter the subarachnoid space, carefully feel for the second, less obvious 'give' as you pierce the dura (the arachnoid mater is closely applied to the under-surface of the dura of the spinal canal).

4. Withdraw the obturator to watch for cerebrospinal fluid emerging from the needle.

Pericardiocentesis

Pericardiocentesis (G *kentesis* = puncture) should be performed with electrocardiographic monitoring.

1. Insert the needle, connected through a three-way tap to a capacious syringe, just to the left of the xiphisternum, aimed towards the tip of the left scapula. Be sensitive to the 'give' as you puncture the pericardium, then aspirate to draw fluid into the syringe.

2. If you irritate the myocardium by contact with the needle you will provoke cardiac irregularities.

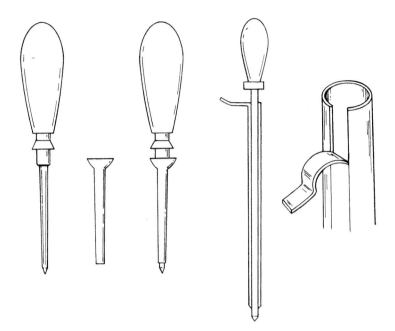

Fig. 4.4 On the left is shown a traditional trocar, then a cannula, and then the trocar fitted into the cannula. On the right is a cross-section of a disposable Lawrence-type trocar and cannula, together with a close-up view of the thin panel being stripped along the length of the cannula so that it can be detached from the catheter that has been inserted through it.

Suprapubic cystostomy

This is an example of the value of distending a tube or cavity in order to enter it. A traditional method is to use a trocar (F *trois* = three + *carré* = side, since the sharp tip of the internal perforator was three-sided) and cannula (Fig. 4.4).

1. Carry it out with strict sterile precautions.

2. Ensure that the bladder is full, confirmed by displaying suprapubic dullness to percussion. Bladder distension peels the peritoneal reflection from bladder wall to abdominal wall upwards, and so avoids the risk of puncturing the peritoneal cavity (Fig. 4.5).

3. Infiltrate the skin with local anaesthetic in the midline, 3–5 cm above the symphysis pubis. Using a longer needle, inject down to and into the bladder wall. When there is a sudden 'give' and you can aspirate urine, you have entered the bladder. Do not continue unless you have confirmed this.

4. Withdraw the syringe and needle. Make a short incision with a scalpel at the site of needle entry and carefully cut vertically down to the bladder wall.

5. Gently insert the trocar and close-fitting cannula along the prepared track and through the bladder wall into the lumen. Avoid sudden uncontrolled penetration that might endanger pelvic structures.

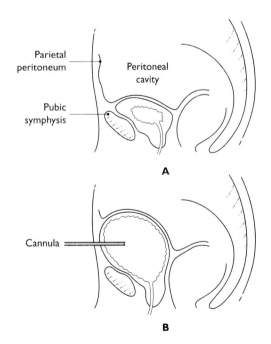

Fig. 4.5 Suprapubic cystostomy. In **A** the bladder is empty. A cannula inserted into the bladder is at risk of transgressing the peritoneal cavity. In **B** the bladder is full and the peritoneal reflexion from the anterior abdomen on to the bladder is well above the track of the cannula.

6. Withdraw the trocar, at which point urine should emerge. Immediately insert a Foley catheter through the cannula.

7. When you are confident that the tip and balloon are in the bladder, carefully remove the cannula without displacing the catheter and inflate the catheter-retaining balloon. A traditional cannula may resist being withdrawn over the bulky catheter outlet. The disposable plastic Lawrence cannula has a detachable strip so that it can be opened out to detach it after withdrawing it from the bladder.

8. Attach the catheter to a drainage tube emptying into a collecting bag. The wound requires only a simple, temporary dressing.

Chest drain

A chest drain allows you to remove air or liquid to achieve and maintain lung expansion (see Ch. 11).

 Key point

- Do not wait to insert a chest drain in the presence of tension pneumothorax. Use needles or a simple incision to release the tension, converting it to a simple pneumothorax.

Peritoneal lavage

Peritoneal lavage through a catheter offers a valuable method of determining whether or not there is intra-abdominal damage.

1. Pass a urinary catheter and nasogastric tube to ensure that the bladder and stomach are empty.

2. Under sterile conditions, after infiltrating local anaesthetic, make a 2 cm vertical incision at the junction of the upper third and lower two-thirds of the line joining the umbilicus and symphysis pubis, into the peritoneal cavity.

3. Insert a finger to ensure that you have safely entered the abdomen and pass in the end of a dialysis catheter, guiding it down towards the pelvis.

4. Alternatively, make a small skin incision and hold up the abdominal wall while carefully inserting a needle carrying an external cannula

into the peritoneal cavity. Attach a syringe and aspirate; if you obtain frank blood do not proceed with lavage.

5. If you do not obtain blood, withdraw the needle and pass in a Seldinger guide wire (see Ch. 5, p. 85), deflecting it towards the pelvis. Withdraw the cannula and insert a catheter over the Seldinger wire.

6. Connect the tube to a container of Ringer's/lactate solution, 10 ml/kg body weight, warmed to body temperature, and slowly run it into the abdomen (Sydney Ringer, 1835–1910, was an English physiologist).

7. Gently agitate the abdomen, wait for 10 minutes, then lower the container to the floor, allowing the fluid to siphon back into the bag. Send a specimen for microscopy.

8. The test is positive if there are more than 100 000 red cells and more than 500 white blood cells per cubic millimetre.

DIRECT INTUBATION

- Ducts, tubes, and spaces that open on to the surface, or are exposed at operation, can be intubated directly.
- By special techniques, internal ducts may be cannulated through instruments such as endoscopes, which are usually passed into hollow viscera via natural orifices; examples are the cannulation of the common bile duct or pancreatic duct through a fibreoptic upper gastrointestinal endoscope, and the catheterization of the ureter through a cystoscope. I shall not describe these since they require special training.
- Plastic, latex rubber, metal and, in the past, gum elastic and other types of catheter have been used with plain open ends, side holes and straight or curved tips (Fig. 4.6). Choose one that slips in easily without being gripped by the walls or you will lose the 'feel' of the catheter. Ducts that can be directly intubated include the trachea, urethra, upper and lower gastrointestinal tract, salivary ducts, stomas, external sinuses and fistulas, or ducts exposed at operation.

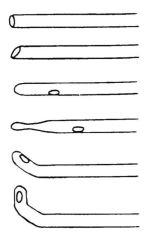

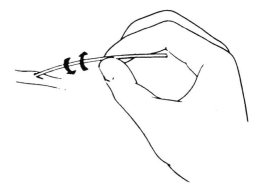

Fig. 4.7   Twist the catheter back and forth between thumb and forefinger to allow it to search out the channel.

Fig. 4.6   Catheter tips. From top to bottom: open end, flute tip, round end with side hole, olivary tip, coudé and bicoudé (F = bent and double-bent).

Key point

- If you have difficulty in advancing a tube or catheter through a convoluted space, do not use force; slightly withdraw it and rotate it before gently advancing it again (Fig. 4.7). In case of difficulty, twist a flexible catheter back and forth between finger and thumb to allow it to search out the channel. When possible, apply gentle traction to straighten the channel.

Tracheal intubation

Tracheal intubation can be carried out through the mouth or through the nose, although nasal intubation requires special skill. You will normally pass an endotracheal tube only on a deeply unconscious patient.

1. Choose an endotracheal tube of the correct length and diameter and test the inflatable cuff.

2. Place the patient supine with a small cushion under the shoulders. Keep the neck straight in the line of the body, slightly flexed, with the head extended at the atlanto-occipital joint, resting on a small pillow.

3. The path the tube will take is a curved one but you must control it under direct vision; this entails temporarily straightening it. Achieve this by using a Mackintosh laryngoscope held in the non-dominant hand.

4. The mouth and opening of the larynx lie anteriorly but the base of the tongue and epiglottis bulge posteriorly. Lift them, and the mandible, by placing the 'beak' of the laryngoscope in the vallecula (L diminutive of *vallis* = valley) between the tongue base and the epiglottis, and gently raise them.

5. You can now look from the head of the table along one or other side of the nose and view the pharynx and laryngeal opening (Fig. 4.8).

6. Pass the tube of correct diameter, length and curvature, under vision, through the laryngeal

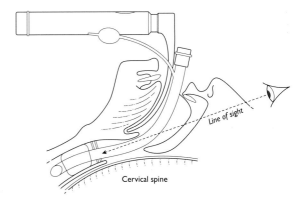

Fig. 4.8   Insertion of an endotracheal tube. The base of the tongue and epiglottis are raised with Mackintosh's laryngoscope. You may look past one side of the nose and the mouth to see the laryngeal opening. The curved endotracheal tube can now be inserted under vision.

opening into the trachea.. The inflatable cuff must lie beyond the vocal cords; gently expand it through the side tube just enough to completely fill the trachea.

7. Check the pressure in the cuff by feeling the small monitor balloon on the inflation tube, then clamp the tube. Collapse of this balloon warns you if the cuff leaks and deflates.

8. Now check that if the chest is compressed air is ejected through the endotracheal tube; if the tube is connected to a bag, which is then compressed, the chest should expand – but ensure that the tube does not lie in the oesophagus by excluding upper abdominal distension or a tympanitic note on percussion.

Feeding jejunostomy

A feeding jejunostomy is an example of a catheter introduced through the abdominal wall at operation, then into the side of the intestine.

1. Place a large haemostat or tissue forceps on the wound edge. Make a stab incision through the abdominal wall in the left upper quadrant of the abdomen well clear of the umbilicus and the rib margin. Evert the wound edge and pass a haemostat through the stab wound from within out, to grasp the tip of the catheter and draw it into the abdomen.

2. Make a small incision in the antimesenteric border of the upper jejunum and pass in approximately 10 cm of tube. Encircle the entry hole with a purse-string suture and tie this, leaving a hole just large enough to insert the catheter, then invert the side wall around the tube with one or more purse-string sutures, creating an ink-well effect.

3. Leave the purse-string suture ends long and take them back and forth around the emerging catheter (see below), tying them to hold it in place. After everting the abdominal wall, insert three or four stitches, each one catching the jejunum close to the emerging catheter and the parietal peritoneum near the stab wound in the abdominal wall. Place all the stitches, then gently tighten them to draw the jejunum into contact with the abdominal wall, forming a seal.

4. After closing the abdominal wall, place a stitch through the skin near the emerging catheter, tie it,

then encircle the catheter and tie it again so that any traction on the catheter does not displace it but is taken by the stitch.

Urethral catheterization

Urethral catheterization in the male is a classical example of the art because it demands great sensitivity, gentleness and skill.

1. Carry out the procedure under strict sterile precautions. Check that you have available an appropriate catheter (e.g. 16–18 F) with the inner sterile plastic container opened but the catheter unexposed, a local anaesthetic tube of 2% lignocaine hydrochloride and sterile nozzle, forceps, towels, swabs, mild aqueous antiseptic solution, water-soluble lubricant, urine receptacle, tubing and collecting bag. Have a syringe and sterile fluid available if you are inserting a Foley-type catheter.

2. Place the patient supine, thighs separated, pudenda exposed. With a sterile swab held in your non-dominant hand grasp the loose dorsal skin of the penis just behind the corona. With another swab held in your dominant hand, push back the uncircumcised foreskin to expose and swab clean the head and corona.

3. Hold up the penis and apply sterile towels – usually a single disposable sheet with a hole in the middle. Replace your grasp with a fresh swab folded lengthwise as a sling that can be held, together with a fold of loose dorsal skin, just behind the corona, between finger and thumb of the non-dominant hand (Fig. 4.9), leaving the other fingers free. Again swab the meatus and penile head with antiseptic solution. Insert the anaesthetic through the nozzle and occlude the urethra to retain it for at least 2 minutes by compressing the under surface of the penis through the sling-like swab, using the medial fingers of your non-dominant hand.

4. Draw the penis vertically upwards, thus straightening the penile urethra (Fig. 4.10). Manipulate the opened inner sterile plastic catheter container to allow 5–7 cm of the tip to protrude. Do not touch the catheter but hold and control it through the cover. Lubricate and insert the catheter tip gently and slowly. Progressively draw back the plastic container.

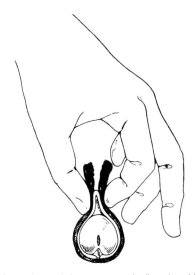

Fig. 4.9 Grasp the penis in a gauze swab sling placed just proximal to the corona. Grip the swab and a fold of loose dorsal skin between finger and thumb, leaving the other fingers free to wrap around the penis to compress the urethra during catheterization to prevent the catheter from being extruded.

5. Prevent the catheter from being extruded following each advancement by wrapping the free fingers of the left hand around the ventral surface covered by the enfolding sterile swab and compressing the urethra against the catheter. The catheter sometimes passes through the sphincter into the bladder if you are patient.

6. If the catheter is held up, draw the penis towards the feet. Without losing your grip on it, swing the penis down between the separated thighs. This has the effect of directing the tip of the catheter upwards into the prostatic urethra and bladder.

7. Ensure that the catheter can empty into a container. Now gently advance it through the prostatic urethra into the bladder. Success is signalled by the appearance of urine. If no urine emerges when the catheter seems to be fully inserted, try pressing on the bladder suprapubically through the sterile towel. Maintain compression of the urethra to prevent the catheter from being extruded until you have secured it.

8. Obtain a specimen of urine for microscopy and culture, then connect the catheter to a closed collecting bag.

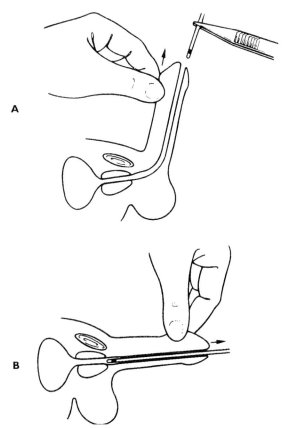

Fig. 4.10 **A** Hold the shaft of the penis dorsally, just behind the corona. First pull it vertically to straighten the penile urethra while you insert the catheter as far as the bulb. **B** Now draw the penis down towards the feet to align the penile and membranous parts of the urethra.

FIXING CATHETERS AND TUBES

Various tubes fulfil an important and sometimes life-saving function. Make sure that you fix them securely and safely. Replacing a catheter that has been inserted with great difficulty and has now fallen out, is challenging – both for you and the patient.

Self-retaining catheters
1. In the past rubber catheters were moulded with projections that could be straightened by stretching or compressing during insertion but they have been largely superseded by the invention of the American urologist Frederic Foley of Minnesota (1891–1966), which is an inflatable balloon near the tip of the

catheter (Fig. 4.11); the catheter can be withdrawn easily after deflating the balloon. A useful retaining device within a small duct is the 'T'-tube catheter (Fig. 4.12). The short limb of the 'T' lies in the duct and allows fluid to flow through it or out of the long limb. When the tube is to be removed, apply gentle traction on the long limb and the flexible cross-pieces of the short limb fold together so that it can be pulled out. The minor leakage dries up rapidly unless there is distal obstruction, and this can be excluded beforehand by radiology following injection of contrast medium.

2. The ability to mould curves in plastic tubes creates a simple means of retaining them. Introduce a pig-tailed catheter after first inserting into it a straight guide wire; withdraw the guide wire, enabling it to regain its natural shape. A double pigtailed catheter (Fig. 4.13), resists movement in either direction, yet when pulled from either end is sufficiently flexible to be withdrawn easily.

Non-self-retaining catheters

1. To retain a catheter indefinitely within a narrow duct, secure it with a ligature or suture–ligature encircling the duct and catheter (Fig. 4.14); the ligature will eventually cut through the wall of the duct. It is difficult to retain a small catheter within the cut end of a wide-bore duct while preventing leakage; try entering the catheter at one side then closing the remaining duct lumen with stitches.

2. Catheters emerging through the skin can be fixed to prevent them from being dislodged in a number of ways (Fig. 4.15). Adhesive plaster or tape may suffice. A stitch inserted through the skin and the tube is a secure method but allows leakage through the stitch hole in the tube. Alternatively, place a stitch through the skin and then lace it back and forth around the tube – so-called 'English lacing', after the manner in which the ancient Britons wrapped their lower legs.

3. An elastic catheter can be neatly fixed by a method shown me by my colleague Miss Phyllis George; cut a small segment from the open end of the tube and stretch it to fit over the emerging catheter. Insert a skin stitch incorporating the cuff that does not pierce the emerging catheter.

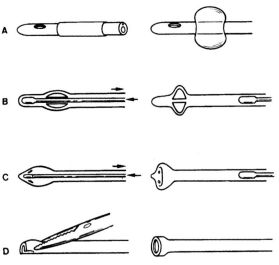

Fig. 4.11 Self-retaining catheters. **A** Foley catheter with an inflatable balloon. **B** De Pezzer and **C** Malecot catheters, both inserted after stretching over an introducer. **D** Winsbury White catheter, inserted with the end folded.

Fig. 4.12 Using a soft, flexible T-tube as a self-retaining catheter. In **A**, it is being inserted through a side hole into the duct. In **B**, the short limb of the 'T' lies in the lumen. It does not obstruct the lumen and allows contents to pass through it or into the long limb. **C** Traction causes the short limbs to come together in order to be pulled out. Any leak rapidly dries up.

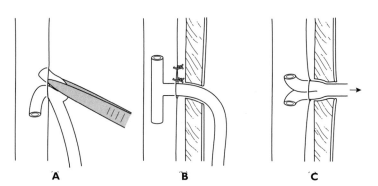

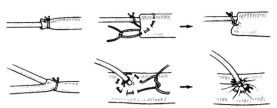

Fig. 4.14 Fixing catheters into small ducts on the left and into larger ducts on the right.

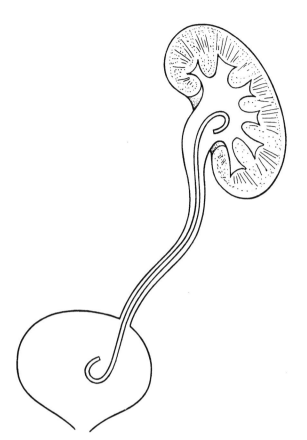

Fig. 4.13 A double pigtailed catheter lies in the ureter. One end is curled in the pelvis of the ureter, the other is curled in the bladder. It may be retrieved easily after grasping the tip within the bladder through a cystoscope.

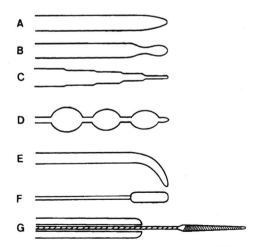

Fig. 4.15 **A** Methods of fixing catheters to the skin using adhesive plaster or stitches. **B** Method suggested by Miss Phyllis George, using a collar cut from the catheter, slipped over it and stitched to the skin.

Bougies

1. Bougies (F = candle, from the town in Algeria where they were made) are usually rods or tubes of circular cross-section (Fig. 4.16) with expanded sections that dilate the channel through which they pass. They may be of rigid or malleable metal, semi-rigid plastic or gum elastic. Dilators may be straight or curved. Metal instruments introduced into the urethra or uterus to probe or dilate the passage are often termed 'sounds' (F *sonder* = to prove, to try).

2. Rigid instruments are damaging in clumsy hands but, when used skilfully, give a better 'feel' and the direction can be controlled. Malleable

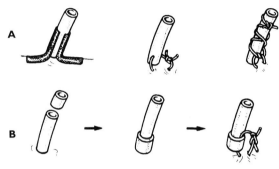

Fig. 4.16 Bougies. **A** Tapered. **B** Olivary-tipped. **C** Stepped. **D** Multiple olives. **E** Curved rigid. **F** Malleable. **G** Hollow dilator threaded over flexible guide wire.

instruments are useful if the shape of the track is irregular.

3. The tip of a dilator is rounded and of smaller diameter than the shank, the transition being gradual. Once the tip has entered the stricture, advancing the instrument gradually dilates it. An olivary-tipped dilator has an oval globular end, likened to an olive; as the olive slips through the stricture its onward passage suddenly becomes easier, providing an estimate of the length of the narrowing – confirmed if necessary by withdrawing it again and noting when the grip of the stricture is suddenly relaxed. The freedom of the dilator after the olive has passed though the narrowing allows you to retain the 'feel' of the passage beyond. As you advance the dilator, it gradually expands the lumen.

4. Start with the largest dilator that is likely to pass, especially if you are using a rigid instrument, since fine rigid instruments too easily perforate the walls of the channel, which may be diseased and fragile.

5. When appropriate, apply a sterile lubricant such as liquid paraffin or a water-soluble jelly.

6. If possible, straighten the channel by exerting traction so there is minimal friction with the walls and you do not lose the 'feel' of the tip. This is possible when you dilate the male urethra.

7. Try varying the direction of the tip until it engages; if this fails, try successively smaller instruments.

8. Multiple strictures require great sensitivity of touch to negotiate them. The grip of each stricture or of a tight orifice dulls your sense of 'feel' for the tip within the next stricture. For this reason dilate each stricture as far as possible before tackling the next one, so that the dilator lies freely until it is gripped by the new stricture.

9. False passages develop when the tip of the dilator enters into side channels opening into the main channel, or into a cul-de-sac created by previous rough instrumentation. Withdraw the dilator and advance it once more while you keep the tip pressed against the opposite wall. It is suggested that one dilator can be left in the false passage to block its mouth while a second instrument passes

along the main duct. I have never succeeded with this method.

10. A filiform (L *filum* = thread, hence threadlike) flexible bougie may be induced to follow a tortuous path through the stricture. If it passes through, a dilator can be screwed to it and guided by it through the stricture; the flexibility of the filiform leader allows it to fold upon itself (Fig. 4.17).

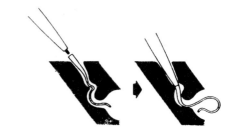

Fig. 4.17 Using a filiform leader as a pilot for the dilator.

Guide wires

1. **Seldinger's wire** (see Ch. 5) is a useful method of following a tortuous channel and negotiating a difficult stricture. Pass the flexible-tipped guide wire through the stricture by gently rotating it back and forth as you advance it through the stricture. Radiographic monitoring of the progress of the tip of the radio-opaque guide wire is invaluable. You may be able to introduce contrast medium to outline the passage. When you have succeeded in advancing the guide wire through the stricture, thread over it a dilator that has a central hole and gently advance this down to, and through, the stricture (Fig. 4.16G). At intervals ensure that the guide wire moves freely within the dilator; fixation of the guide wire indicates that it is trapped and kinked so the tip of the dilator is not entering the stricture and could perforate the side wall of the duct.

11. When you can pass an endoscope down to a stricture, you may be able to negotiate a guide wire through it under vision, as in the oesophagus. You can leave the guide wire in place, remove the endoscope and pass graded dilators with a central channel over the guide wire to dilate the stricture.

12. Occasionally it is impossible to pass even a fine guide wire through. In some circumstances, if one end of a thread is fixed proximally and the other

end is introduced above the stricture, this will eventually be carried through by fluid flow and by peristalsis. After retrieving the distal end, attach a thin, flexible dilator to the proximal end. Exert slight traction on the distal thread to guide and draw through the tip of the fine dilator (Fig. 4.18). I have used this method, devised by Mr Richard Franklin, with success in overcoming seemingly impassable oesophageal strictures.

13. Commonly, you can pass a series of graduated dilators, each one being slightly thicker than the previous one. As you negotiate the stricture, note the details of the passage. Do not remove it until you have the next dilator ready. Now smoothly draw out the first dilator and immediately and gently slide in the next size, and so on. The tip of each bigger dilator is slightly smaller than the shank of its predecessor. Control the direction of insertion and passage of a rigid dilator by movement of the handle (Fig. 4.19). A rigid, curved dilator cannot be rotated while it lies in a narrow channel but if it reaches a wider channel it can be rotated. Confirm that you

have reached the bladder by this method when dilating urethral strictures.

14. Sometimes, natural channels require dilatation, as a rule only as the result of damage or disease with stricture formation. Occasionally you may need to gently stretch a normal channel in order to insert instruments or substances.

> ## 🔑 Key points
>
> - Never use force to drive the tip of the dilator through the stricture. Misdirected force creates a false passage that will abort future attempts.
> - It is better to stretch a stricture than to tear it. Tearing, usually signalled by bleeding, results in further fibrosis; as fibrous tissue matures it contracts and re-forms the stricture. Do not be too ambitious – be willing to stop before you achieve the maximum diameter, and repeat the procedure at increasing intervals, gaining a little each time.
> - Never fail to record the size of the dilators and details of the peculiarities of the passage on each occasion, for future guidance.

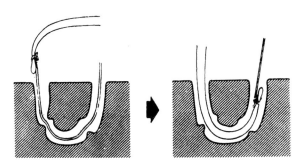

Fig. 4.18 A thread has been induced to pass the stricture and acts as a leader for the dilator.

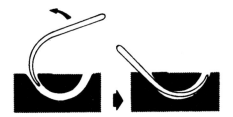

Fig. 4.19 Negotiating a curved channel with a rigid curved dilator. The handle of the dilator must be swung in an arc to direct the point along the curved path.

Balloons

- When a dilator is pushed through a stricture there is a damaging shear force on the duct lining. As this heals, scar tissue is laid down, contracts as it matures, recreating the stricture. When possible, avoid the shearing force by exerting centrifugal distension from within the stricture. An excellent method of achieving this is by balloon dilatation.
- Over-distension of the balloon may disrupt the wall; for this reason balloons are available that reach a predetermined maximum diameter then rupture if over-inflated.

1. Negotiate a collapsed balloon across the stricture and inflate it, exerting only radial forces (Fig. 4.20). The balloons can be passed under vision, mounted on catheters threaded over guide wires, or over endoscopes. They can be accurately placed under radiological control and for this reason they usually incorporate radio-opaque markers.

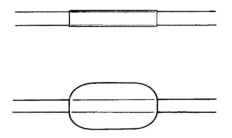

Fig. 4.20   The catheter carries a collapsed balloon, which can be placed within a stricture. When the balloon is inflated it exerts a radial dilating effect.

2. Balloon dilatation is sometimes used to overstretch the sphincteric muscles of, for example, the lower oesophagus to overcome a hold-up resulting from achalasia (G *a* = not + *chalasis* = relaxation).

Other methods

1. Dilators that expand while they lie within a narrow channel have been used for many years. A classic method is a laminaria tent (L *tenta* = a probe) in which a cylinder of dried seaweed is inserted in a duct; as it absorbs water it expands and dilates the channel. The method has long been in use to dilate the uterine cervical canal to procure an abortion.

2. Mechanical expansile dilatation from within the lumen can be used to dilate stenosed heart valves.

3. One type of stent can be sited in a stricture and then expanded by inflating a balloon within it; the stent then holds its shape.

4. Special materials have been developed in the last few years in order to produce wire mesh elastic expanders. The mesh is compressed to produce a long thin tube that is released when it lies across the narrowing. It actively adopts a shorter and wider shape that expands the narrowed segment, or is sometimes passively expanded using an inflatable balloon (see Fig. 4.44, p. 65).

5. When the lumen of a duct is encroached on by an ingrowth of diseased tissue such as cancer, the passage can often be restored using several forms of treatment including radiotherapy, laser therapy and chemotherapy.

ENDOSCOPIC ACCESS

- Endoscopy and 'down the line of sight' operative procedures have been well established for many years through an extensive range of rigid and flexible endoscopes.
- Instruments can be inserted into natural tubes and manoeuvred by 'feel.'
- The advances were possible because of improvements in visualization and instrumentation.
- Improvements in imaging reduce the need for physical exploration.
- A wide range of instruments can be introduced through open tubes or through special channels in more sophisticated endoscopes (G *endon* = within + *skopeein* = to view), with good lighting and visual characteristics, into natural or abnormal channels, including catheters, dilators, balloons, diathermy wires, forceps, scissors, cytology brushes, Dormier baskets and snares (Fig. 4.21).
- Instruments with moving parts such as scissors, forceps and snares can be activated by two rods sliding on each other, or one rod sliding within a rigid tube; the moving rod can be pushed or pulled. Flexible instruments often employ the principle of the Bowden cable – the mechanism for controlling most bicycle brakes. The inner wire can be pulled but not pushed; if the inner wire has been pulled within the flexible tube, release must be by some distal spring action.
- Handle designs vary but all rely on a gripping motion or separation of the hand or of a finger and thumb (Fig. 4.22). Because the tissues cannot be held and steadied while they are being cut with scissors, the blades may advantageously be claw-shaped (Fig. 4.21), to prevent the tissue from sliding away.

1. When introducing a rigid instrument along a convoluted channel, be extremely sensitive to the hold-ups. Be willing to withdraw it slightly, adjust the angle and gently advance it again. Try to keep the tip of the instrument in the centre of the lumen.

2. If a straight instrument has an angled tip it may be rotated within a flexible but twisting channel to

Fig. 4.21 Some of the instruments that can be used down an endoscope. From top to bottom: catheter, dilator, diathermy wire tightened to produce a 'cheese-cutter' effect, forceps, scissors, cytology brush, Dormier basket and a snare.

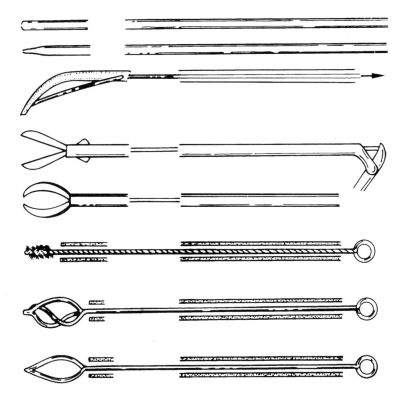

Fig. 4.22 Methods of controlling moving tipped instruments. **A** A wire passes through a spiral wire flexible tube. This Bowden cable mechanism can be pulled but not pushed. **B** A rigid system of a rod passing through a metal tube. This allows both pulling and pushing.

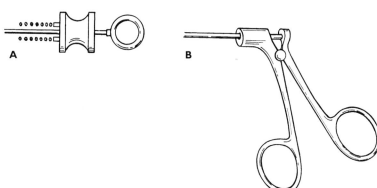

assist the progress of its tip. A classic example is the shape of a cystoscope through the male urethra. Once the angled tip of the cystoscope enters the bladder cavity it can be rotated and moved – the shaft has straightened the urethra (Fig. 4.23).

3. Of necessity, rigid instruments passed under vision must be manoeuvred along the line of sight. Depth perception is limited. The point of action of instruments with an offset tip can be controlled by rotating them.

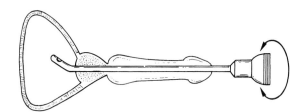

Fig. 4.23 A bent but flexible duct such as a male urethra can be straightened. The angled tip of the instrument follows the bends of the urethra because it can be rotated. Once it enters the bladder the tip can be freely rotated and advanced or withdrawn.

4. Flexible instruments are difficult to control within a wide channel or open tube but their flexibility may facilitate progression along a tortuous track. However, the tip may engage in an irregularity; if it does, withdraw it slightly, rotate it and gently advance it. Remember, there is less 'feel' with a flexible instrument than with a rigid one.

5. An instrument or catheter can be led out of a tube through a side hole to angulate it (Fig. 4.24). Some rigid and flexible endoscopes have a controllable lever to vary the angle of emergence. This was originally designed by the Parisian urologist of Cuban origin, Jacques Albarran (1860–1912). The tip of the instrument or tube can be kept in view through a side-viewing telescope.

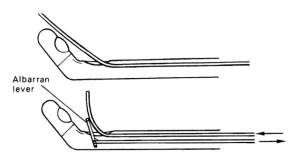

Fig. 4.24 A flexible catheter or instrument can be passed out of the side of a rigid or flexible endoscope. The angle of emergence can be controlled using an Albarran lever.

RIGID INSTRUMENTS

- The **cystoscope** was one of the first endoscopic instruments to reach a very high standard of development. Through it, you may inspect the bladder, take biopsies, fulgurate tumours and catheterize ureters. Fibreoptic cystoscopes can be passed relatively painlessly.
- Transurethral resection of the prostate gland can be achieved using a diathermy loop, through a resectoscope. Urethroscopy, ureteroscopy and percutaneous nephrostomy can be carried out.

 Key point

- Safe passage of instruments for the various forms of single access to tubes and spaces requires specialized training, especially in order to interpret the findings and perform procedures that sometimes require skills at the limits of technical accomplishment. Some procedures, such as laryngoscopy, proctoscopy and sigmoidoscopy, should be well within the capability of any surgical trainee. Take every opportunity to learn how to use these endoscopes effectively.

Sigmoidoscopy

Rigid sigmoidoscopy provides on a larger scale the opportunity to practise gentle, skilful manipulation of a tube.

1. Place the patient on the left side, buttocks overhanging the right side of the couch, knees drawn up to the chest, feet on the far side from you as you stand on the right side of the couch (Fig. 4.25).

 Key point

- Never insert an endoscope without first inspecting the perianal area and carrying out a careful digital examination, after explaining to the patient what you are doing.

2. Gently place the tip of the obturator within the well-lubricated sigmoidoscope (Fig. 4.26) against the patient's anus, pointing towards the umbilicus. Maintain only slight pressure until the sphincter relaxes, allowing you to insert the sigmoidoscope for about 6–8 cm, when it abuts against the anterior wall of the rectum. Hold the sigmoidoscope steady while you withdraw the obturator and fit on the viewing end seal with attached light bulb and air pump.

3. Perform all subsequent manoeuvres under vision. Insufflate only sufficient air to separate the walls and allow you to guide the endoscope safely without causing discomfort. You are now close up to the anterior rectal wall. To regain the view of the

Fig. 4.25 Sigmoidoscopy, seen from above. The sigmoidoscope is angled after initial insertion to view the rectum, which lies in the hollow of the sacrum.

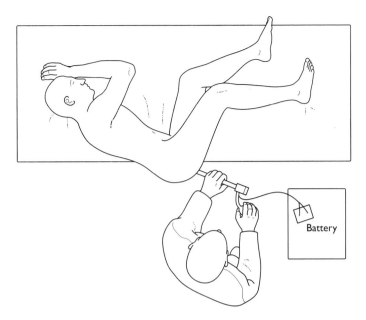

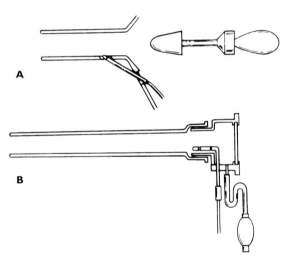

Fig. 4.26 **A** A short proctoscope, which is an open hollow tube. The obturator has been withdrawn. **B** A rigid sigmoidoscope, which is an open tube that can be closed off so the bowel can be inflated and distended. The cap has a transparent window.

lumen you need to swing the outer end of the endoscope anteriorly to turn the internal portion into the rectum lying in the hollow of the sacrum. Concentrate initially on introducing the instrument to the intended limit, keeping the tip centred in the bowel lumen. As you withdraw it in a spiral manner you can examine every part of the interior, paying particular attention to the mucosa and any abnormalities.

4. If you wish to remove a biopsy or swab specimen, you must remove the viewing end and allow the air to escape. First of all bring your objective into the centre of view; usually you can trap it by enclosing it and gently pressing the tip of the instrument against the bowel wall. Do not overinflate the rectum or it will suddenly deflate and the target mucosa will move. Insert the biopsy forceps or swab and obtain the specimen, then replace the viewing end-piece so that you can reinflate the rectum and complete the examination.

5. Deflate the rectum and warn the patient as you finally withdraw the sigmoidoscope, since it feels like an embarrassing defecation.

Proctoscopy

Proctoscopy is carried out in a similar manner, but retain the obturator until you have fully introduced the instrument. Once more, remember that you must swing the handle portion forward on the patient to negotiate the almost 90º angle between anus and rectum. Only now should you remove the obturator.

1. Carefully view the interior of the lower rectum and anal canal as you slowly withdraw the proctoscope.

2. As the rim of the proctoscope descends in the anal canal the sphincter attempts to extrude it and you need to apply slight pressure to prevent this while you examine the lower anal canal.

Haemorrhoid injection

Injection of haemorrhoids with sclerosant must be directed into the perivascular tissues around the upper pole of each pile.

1. During your first introduction and withdrawal of the proctoscope take careful note of the situation of the haemorrhoids as they prolapse over the lip of the withdrawing endoscope. Traditionally they were recorded as though the patient lay supine in the lithotomy position at 4, 7 and 11 o'clock related to a clock face. Since the patient now usually lies on the left side, they are usually at 1, 4 and 8 o'clock.

2. As you withdraw the proctoscope until the piles prolapse into the lumen, they obscure your view of their bases. You must now remove the proctoscope, replace the obturator, fully reintroduce it and remove the obturator.

3. Slowly withdraw the proctoscope until a rim of anus appears and the sphincter begins to extrude the proctoscope. Resist this but angle the proctoscope to reveal a complete ring of about 0.5 cm of anal canal. If the haemorrhoids prolapse you are too low; withdraw the proctoscope, reinsert it and start again.

4. Taking each site in turn, insert the shouldered needle attached to the filled haemorrhoid syringe. Aspirate. If blood enters the syringe you are within the vessel. Fully withdraw the needle and reinsert it in a slightly different site until you cannot aspirate any blood.

5. Inject approximately 5–10 ml of 5% phenol in almond or arachis (peanut) oil into the submucosa at the base of the pile. Watch as you inject. You should produce a slight swelling; if the swelling blanches,

you are too superficial, if there is no swelling you are too deep.

 Key point

- Haemorrhoid injection cannot be performed with a single injection of the proctoscope. Injection must be perivascular, into the base of each pile, and never into the vessel.

Other rigid instruments

Laryngoscopes, auriscopes (L *auris* = ear), colposcopes (G *kolpos* = sinus or pocket, but applied to the vagina), hysteroscope (G *hysteros* = womb), and many other endoscopes are used. In some cases the instrument is called a speculum (L = a mirror, from *spectare* = to look), since a mirror was inserted. Nasal and vaginal specula are in common use.

FLEXIBLE ENDOSCOPES

- Fibreoptic endoscopy became possible following the development of coherent glass fibre bundles by Harold Hopkins in Reading (Fig. 4.27), applied to gastrointestinal endoscopy by Basil Hirschowitz of Birmingham, Alabama.
- A variety of controllable, flexible endoscopes can be passed into the upper and lower gastrointestinal tract (Fig. 4.28), the trachea and bronchi, urinary and gynaecological tracts, and other tubes, blood vessels and spaces.

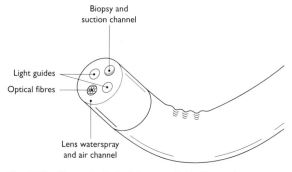

Fig. 4.28 The end of a flexible controllable fibreoptic endoscope, showing the light and optical ports, biopsy and suction channels, the lens water spray and air insufflation channel.

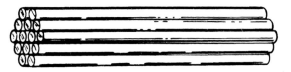

Fig. 4.27 A coherent bundle of glass fibres. They transmit light in a constant relationship within the fibres throughout the bundle.

- The instruments are remarkably versatile and inspection, biopsy, snaring, dilatation, diathermization, the capture, ultrasonic shock and laser beam fragmentation of stones, and other specialized procedures can be carried out with their aid.

DISPLAY

- Some ducts such as the bowel lie free while others, such as intrahepatic bile ducts and bronchi, are buried in connective tissue. Take every opportunity to recognize ducts by gaining an intimate knowledge of the anatomy, appearance and feel. For example, the ureter has a characteristic vermiculating peristalsis. Ducts opening on to a surface, such as the urethra and salivary ducts, can be catheterized to delineate their paths. Fistulous tracks can be followed by inserting a probe or injecting dye.
- Radio-opaque media can be injected through catheters, administered orally or parenterally and may be excreted into ducts to be displayed on X-rays such as cholecystograms and urograms. Other imaging methods may also be used to aid identification and location.

1. When seeking a duct lying in homogeneous tissue, always cut in the expected line of the duct rather than at right angles to it, to avoid the risk of transecting it.

2. If you wish to display a long segment of duct take care not to damage any tributaries or divisions and respect its blood and nervous supply.

3. Remember that a collapsed and empty duct may be imperceptible but can be made more prominent by distending it with fluid or cannulating it.

4. Protect a fragile duct from injury as you display it by separating overlying tissues with care. Gently insert the rounded tips of non-toothed forceps superficial to the duct, allow them to open and cut between the separated blades (Fig. 4.29). Blunt-nosed haemostatic forceps are valuable dissecting instruments when freeing ducts; insinuate the closed blades next to the duct and gently open them parallel to it (Fig. 4.30). If the

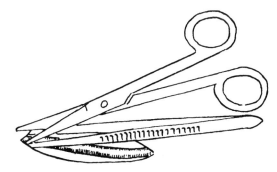

Fig. 4.29 Display a duct by placing dissecting forceps superficial to it, allow the forceps blades to separate, and cut between them.

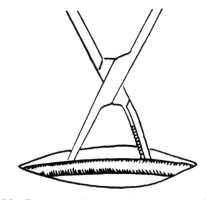

Fig. 4.30 Displaying a duct by opening haemostatic forceps parallel to it.

duct has tributaries, or if it branches, it is sometimes preferable to open the forceps at right angles to the duct (Fig. 4.31).

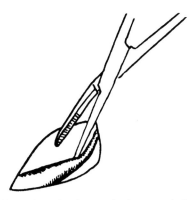

Fig. 4.31 Displaying a duct by opening haemostatic forceps at right angles to it.

OCCLUSION

Divided duct

1. The duct may be divided deliberately or accidentally.

2. Diathermization under compression creates a weld in a small duct but is usually an insecure method of sealing it.

3. If it is important that the channel does not re-form, as when carrying out vasectomy or female sterilization by occluding the fallopian tubes, divide them after doubly ligating or clipping them and separate the ends.

4. Ligation is usually safe and effective but do not tie it too tightly or it may cut right through. Do not apply the ligature too near the end or it may slip off or be gradually rolled off if the duct undergoes peristalsis (Fig. 4.32). As a safeguard against this, insert a transfixion suture–ligature (Fig. 4.33). If spillage of contents is a risk, apply double ligatures before transecting the duct between them (Fig. 4.34).

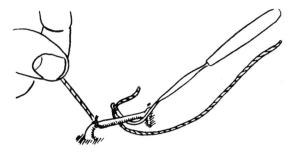

Fig. 4.34 If there is a risk of spillage, do not transect the duct until you have applied two ligatures at a distance from each other, then cut between them.

5. Close a supple large-bore duct using a simple ligature reinforced by invaginating the end within a purse-string suture (Fig. 4.35).

6. Flatten a supple but thicker-walled duct and close it with a linear suture (Fig. 4.36). This can be

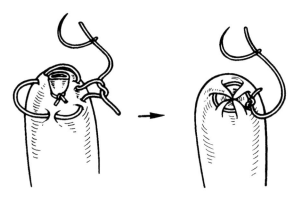

Fig. 4.35 On the left a ligature has been tied to close the end of a large duct. On the right the closed end has been invaginated with a purse string suture.

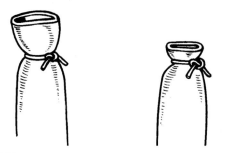

Fig. 4.32 Do not apply ligatures too near the end of a duct. The one on the right may slip off or be rolled off by peristalsis.

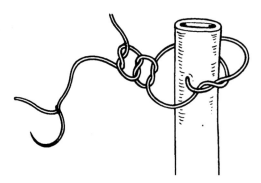

Fig. 4.33 Transfixion suture–ligature. The needled thread has been passed through the duct before being tied.

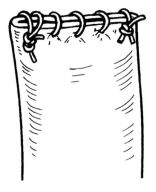

Fig. 4.36 Closing a wide-bore tube with a row of sutures after flattening the end.

reinforced by invaginating it within a second layer of sutures (Fig. 4.37).

7. A single metal or absorbable clip is sufficient to occlude a small duct. Close the flattened end of a larger duct with a linear stapler (Fig. 4.38).

> ### Key point
>
> • When there is a choice, prefer sutures to clips; they are more versatile – and less likely to catch in other tissues, instruments or materials, and be dragged off.

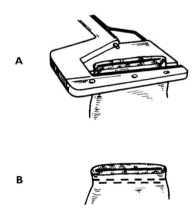

Fig. 4.37 A linear suture-closure (or staple-closure) of a duct can be reinforced by invaginating the first suture line with a second layer of sutures.

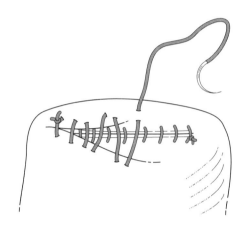

Fig. 4.38 Closing a deformable tube with a double row of staples. **A** Apply the stapler across the duct and actuate it. **B** When the stapler is removed the double line of staples can be seen.

In continuity

If it is unnecessary or undesirable to divide a small, supple duct to occlude the lumen, apply a ligature, or a metal clip. Larger supple tubes cannot be occluded in this manner and must be flattened and closed with a line of stitches or a line of staples.

Control of leakage

1. Achieve temporary control by simple compression, constriction with a thread or tape ligature or apply one of the large variety of non-crushing clamps to occlude the flow of content. The curved Satinsky-type clamp does not obstruct flow along the duct but isolates a potential source of leakage while it is being repaired, joined or closed (Fig. 4.39).

2. Alternatively, occlude the lumen using a balloon obturator such as a Foley catheter, which can be deflated and withdrawn at the last minute before final closure. If necessary, fluid can be introduced into or drained from the duct through the main channel of the catheter.

3. The principle of a cuffed tube is employed when an endotracheal tube is passed to inflate the lungs during anaesthesia or to provide respiratory assistance (Fig. 4.40). Inflate the cuff, lying in the trachea, to prevent leakage around the tube during respiratory inflation.

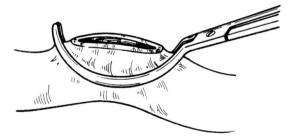

Fig. 4.39 The curved Satinsky-type clamp allows flow along the lower part of the duct as the open upper part is isolated to control leakage.

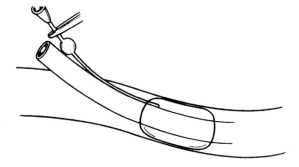

Fig. 4.40 The tube has an external cuff that can be inflated through a side tube. This channels all fluids through the tube lumen. The technique facilitates inflation of the lungs through a cuffed endotracheal tube (see Fig. 4.8, p. 49).

DISOBLITERATION

1. A duct can be blocked as a result of many factors:
- in the lumen, the contents – for example inspissated (L *spissare* = thicken) contents, worms, flukes in the bowel, stones in the ureter, bile duct or salivary duct
- in the wall, for example a stricture, tumour, or failure to transmit the contents by peristalsis
- external factors, as from adhesions, bands, hernial orifices and external tumours
- a combination of these.

> 🔑 **Key point**
>
> - How you manage the blockage depends upon its cause – is it likely to recur? If the cause is progressive, for example malignant obstruction, you need to isolate any corrective procedure from encroachment by the disease.

2. If obstruction results from a stricture it may be dilated. A tumour can be shrunk by external radiotherapy, local irradiation – brachytherapy (G *brachys* = short) – or chemotherapy.

3. Stones can often be pulverized (L *pulvis* = powder) by shock-wave lithotripsy (G *lithos* = stone + *ripsis* = rubbing), ultrasound or laser therapy. Accessible stones can be crushed and, with

other obstructions, can often be removed using forceps or other instruments passed through an endoscope (Fig. 4.41). In some cases disobliteration can be carried out endoscopically either by resection, as in transurethral resection of the prostate, by vaporization with a laser beam, as with oesophageal carcinoma, or by restoring the lumen by inserting a splinting tube (Fig. 4.42). This may be inserted by first dilating the narrow segment and leaving in a bougie, then passing over this a plastic tube advanced through the narrow segment with a 'pusher' tube (Fig. 4.43). Insertion of such tubes often demands immediate and extensive preliminary dilatation. In many sites this can be avoided by inserting a tube stent made of springy metal that can be introduced across the narrowing in a compressed state and allowed to expand spontaneously (Fig. 4.44).

4. It may be necessary to deal with an obstruction by open operation. On occasion non-invasive methods have failed, or are inappropriate. For example, normal or diseased bowel may be obstructed by a swallowed foreign body, impacted

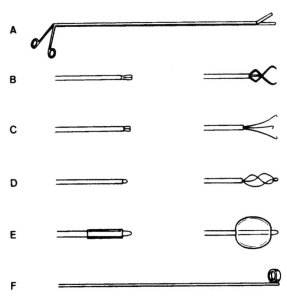

Fig. 4.41 Instruments for removing obstructions. **A** A rigid 'alligator' forceps. **B** and **C** Flexible grasping forceps, shown closed and open. **D** A Dormier basket, shown closed and open. **E** A balloon catheter, shown deflated and inflated. **F** An internal ring stripper.

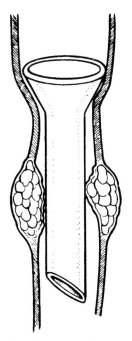

Fig. 4.42 A plastic hollow stent has been impacted in a tube to hold it open. The flared upper end is designed to prevent the stent from passing through the stricture.

food, a gallstone that has ulcerated into the bowel, or a ball of intestinal worms. Do not immediately open the duct. Soft material may be disimpacted, broken up and manoeuvred through a narrow segment and allowed to pass through normally. If this is impossible, consider massaging it proximally and open the duct here where it is less likely to have suffered damage. Remove the cause of the block and carefully repair the opening. This is now rarely required for impacted stones in the ureter, bile ducts or salivary ducts. Especially when removing salivary duct stones, guard against them slipping back into the gland by encircling the duct with a thread or a gently closed tissue forceps, before opening the duct (Fig. 4.45).

5. A narrow segment of a supple duct can be widened by a plastic (G *plassein* = to form) procedure. It was originally devised to overcome strictures resulting from long-standing ulceration at the pylorus and named *pyloroplasty*. It has been adapted for dealing with the small-bowel strictures resulting from *Crohn's inflammatory bowel disease*. Make a longitudinal incision through the full length

Fig. 4.43 The safest way to introduce a stent is to dilate the stricture and leave a bougie within the lumen. Slide the stent over the bougie, using a 'pusher', to advance it into position.

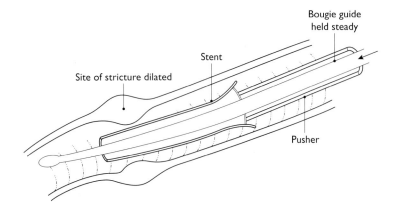

Fig. 4.44 Expanding stent. The springy wire stent is compressed, making it long and thin. When it is correctly placed across the stricture it is released and expands its diameter while shortening its length, expanding the narrow segment.

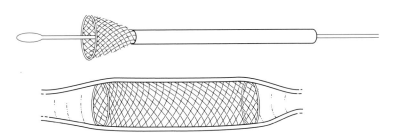

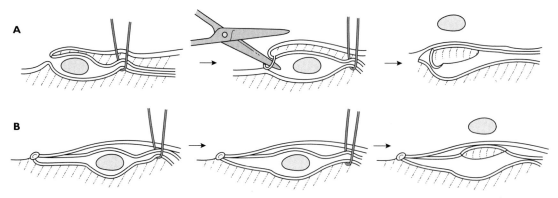

A

B

Fig. 4.45 Removing an obstructing stone from a superficial duct. In **A**, the stone is near the orifice, which can be divided with scissors. In **B**, the stone lies some distance from the orifice. Cut down on it through the overlying epithelium. The stitch encircling the duct prevents the stone from slipping backwards when it is lifted to kink the duct. Gently pull it through after removing the stone.

of the stricture, open it out and close the defect as a transverse suture line (Fig. 4.46).

6. It may be preferable to excise a narrow segment and bring the ends together directly to bridge the defect (Fig. 4.47A). The circumferential suture line that results may narrow the lumen; if so, minimize this by cutting the duct diagonally at each end of the stricture, producing a longer oblique line of closure (Fig. 4.47B).

7. **Immovable or recurrent obstruction** can be dealt with in many ways. You may accept the blockage; an example is blockage of a ureter below a poorly functioning kidney with good function of the other kidney. One method of relief is bypass, creating an internal stoma (G = mouth) with the duct below the obstruction or with another channel, for example draining a blocked bile duct or ureter into the bowel. In some cases the creation of an *external stoma* may be valuable because it allows the output to be measured.

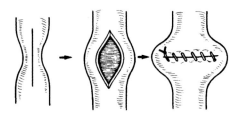

Fig. 4.46 Make a longitudinal incision through the whole length of the stricture. Open it out, draw the two ends together and close the defect as a transverse incision, creating a shorter but wider tube.

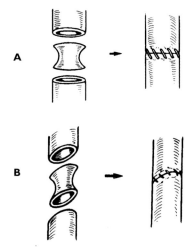

A

B

Fig. 4.47 **A** Excise the stricture and join the cut ends. **B** End-to-end anastomosis with a circumferential suture line may leave a constriction. This can be avoided by cutting the ends obliquely and joining them.

 Key point

- Differentiate between a duct that is merely a conduit and one that secretes or fills with content; for example, the bowel secretes enzymes and mucus. If the duct secretes into the lumen, you must not leave a closed segment or loop, which will become distended with its own secretions.

8. Bypass may be possible without transecting the duct (Fig. 4.48A1). Draw up a distal loop proximally and unite it above the obstruction, to carry on the obstructed contents (Fig. 4.48A2). Contents may stagnate in the segment between the obstruction and the stoma. An external stoma can also be created without transecting the duct (Fig. 4.48A3); again, content may stagnate in the segment between the obstruction and the external stoma.

9. The duct may be transected below the obstruction (Fig. 4.48B1), allowing you to draw up the distal cut end above it (Fig. 4.48B2) and close off the stump below the obstruction. Do not close off the stump if it is likely to become distended; prefer to join the cut end into the draining loop (Fig. 4.48B3) or bring it to the surface (Fig. 4.48B4); this is often termed a draining fistula (L = pipe) to distinguish it from a stoma, which drains the whole duct content.

10. The duct may be transected above an irremovable obstruction (Fig. 4.48C1) and brought to the surface as stoma (Fig. 4.48C2). If a secreting remnant above the obstruction is closed off, it may become filled and rupture. One solution is to create a loop stoma (Fig. 4.48A3) but, to prevent any flow

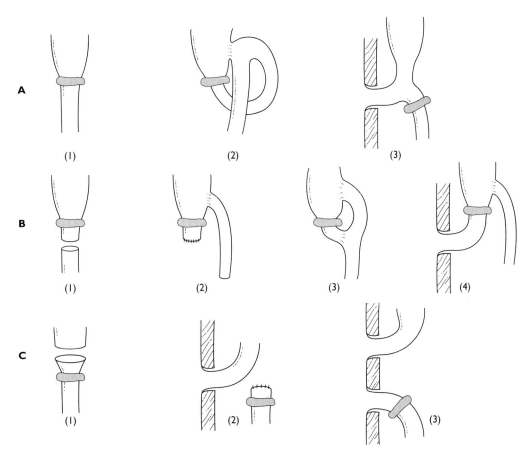

Fig. 4.48 Possibilities for dealing with an irremovable obstruction. **A** (1) Do not transect the obstructed segment above or below the blockage. (2) Draw up a distal loop from beyond the obstruction and form an anastomosis proximal to the obstruction. (3) Bring the segment above the obstruction to the surface to form an external stoma. **B** (1) Transect the distal duct below the obstruction. (2) Draw the lower cut end proximally to unite it above the obstruction. Close off the distal stump beyond the block. (3) If there is a risk of the remnant below becoming distended by local secretions if it is closed, join it into the draining loop or (4) bring it to the surface as a draining fistula. **C** (1) Transect the bowel above the obstruction. (2) Bring out the upper cut end to the surface as a terminal stoma and close the stump above the block. (3) If the closed stump is likely to become distended, bring the stump to the surface as a draining fistula.

down the loop, separate stomata can be created (Fig. 4.48C3), so the proximal duct is drained but also the duct between the distal cut end and the stoma. If you cannot drain the segment internally or bring it to the surface as a stoma, consider inserting a tube to bridge the distance between the loop and the surface (Fig. 4.49). If the tube remains in position for a considerable period, a fistulous track may form so that the contents reach the surface even when the tube is withdrawn.

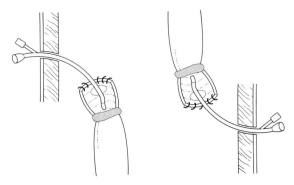

Fig. 4.49 If you need to leave a fixed, closed compartment that may fill up, and which cannot be drained internally, insert a self-retaining catheter. Bring the catheter to the exterior.

REPAIR

Ducts may be damaged accidentally or deliberately – as when performing a surgical manoeuvre to gain access.

 Key point

- To achieve success, carry out the repair perfectly, without tension, on a healthy duct with an adequate blood supply and protect it during the healing phase.

Gastrointestinal tract
1. If the bowel has been injured, assiduously search for every possible blunt or penetrating wound. Check the mesentery for potential threats to the blood supply.

2. The area of the mucosa is far greater than the area of the submucosa and seromuscularis, particularly in the small intestine. When the bowel wall is acutely breached, therefore, the mucosa tends to evert. This brings into apposition the mucosal surfaces, forming a channel for leakage of contents (Fig. 4.50). If it is difficult to replace the mucosa, use an inverting mattress stitch, often referred to in this context as a Connell stitch, after the 19th-century American surgeon who popularised it.

3. In contrast, a breach resulting from chronic ulceration or inflammation is associated with fibrosis that fixes the mucosa, so that it does not protrude. As a rule you can safely bring the margins together with a simple all-coats suture, as in closing a perforated peptic ulcer, although many surgeons include an overlying tag of omentum in the closing stitch.

Other ducts and cavities
1. Because many ducts are of small calibre, repair of defects or injuries may result in a stricture; this becomes more likely if you fail to appose the lining epithelium with every stitch. Make sure to excise all necrotic tissue or the repair will break down. In many cases the best option is re-anastomosis or anastomosis to a large duct such as bowel.

2. Take great care, when mobilizing small ducts, not to damage the blood supply, which is often tenuous (L *tenuis* = thin). For this reason, do not try to free it excessively.

3. Recognize iatrogenic (G *iatros* = physician) injuries and repair them immediately, especially bile ducts and ureter. The pancreatic duct is not usually repaired but drained into the bowel.

4. Repair of the ovarian tubes, vas deferens, salivary and lachrymal ducts demands microsurgical methods (see Ch. 5) in order to preserve or regain tubal patency.

5. Repair of a cavity wall, such as the urinary bladder, is less critical because there is more available tissue. Urologists usually employ stitches that exclude the mucosa – extramucosal stitches. The bladder can contract very powerfully, so it is usual to insert a suprapubic or transurethral catheter to ensure that pressure does not build up.

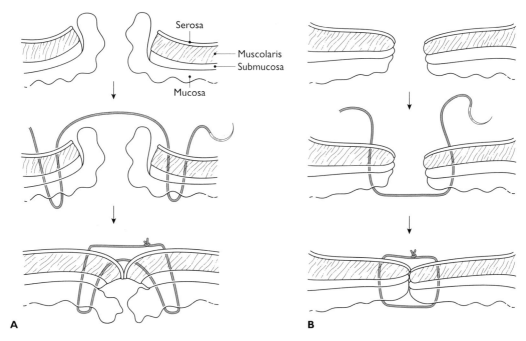

Fig. 4.50 Repair of traumatic rupture of bowel. **A** Section through an acute traumatic puncture of the bowel wall often results in pouting of the mucosa; this can be corrected using an inverting (Connell) mattress suture. **B** A chronic cause has resulted in fibrosis with fixation of the layers; it can be closed using a simple stitch, producing an edge-to-edge union.

ANASTOMOSIS

Galen (AD 131–201) used this term (G *ana* = through + *stoma* = a mouth, hence 'a coming together through a mouth'). Ducts of the same or different types can be joined together.

Obey the important rules when performing anastomoses of ducts:

- Ducts of all types must retain or gain an adequate arterial blood supply and venous drainage, in order to heal.
- Ensure that the anastomosis is performed between disease-free ducts. Inflammation, infection, neoplasms or foreign bodies all threaten healing.
- Do not join ducts without excluding distal obstruction.
- Some ducts, notably the bowel, have autonomous directional peristalsis. If you forget this, drainage of the contents may be impaired.
- Ensure that there is no tension, no twisting or excessive constriction when ducts are joined.

- Avoid back pressure and stagnation; bacteria rapidly flourish in stagnant contents.

BOWEL

 Key points

- Stitching remains the most versatile method of joining bowel; while you are training take every opportunity to practise. Use stapling techniques only when they offer distinct benefits.
- Use non-toothed dissecting forceps, preferably to apply counterpressure and gently deform the tissues rather than to grasp and crush the delicate bowel wall.
- Do not rush to start. 'Set up' the procedure by first arranging the bowel so that you can perform the anastomosis in the most natural manner possible.
- Should you change your own position, perhaps go to the other side of the operating table?

1. Ensure that the bowel ends match. If they do not, be willing to angle the end of the narrower end, to enlarge it. Cut back on the edge opposite the entrance of the blood supply – the antimesenteric edge (Fig. 4.51).

2. You may apply non-crushing bowel clamps to steady the ends and prevent leakage of content. Alternatively, insert traction sutures at each end (Fig. 4.52). If you need to suture the back wall first when the bowel cannot be rotated, insert the traction sutures just posterior to the junction of the back and front walls, so that the anterior walls remain slack when the sutures are distracted, allowing easy access to the back wall. Some surgeons distract the middle of the anterior walls with traction sutures or tissue forceps while they insert stitches in the back wall.

3. Types of stitch are determined by your beliefs, training and current fashion, since no satisfactory controlled trials have been carried out comparing popular methods. The strongest and therefore most important layer to include is the submucous, collagenous coat – the coat from which catgut is

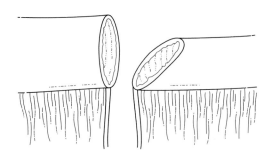

Fig. 4.51 If the ends are disparate in calibre, cut back the narrower end on the side opposite the mesentery or the entry of the blood supply.

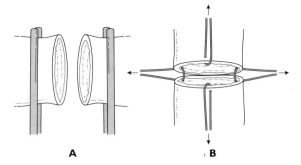

A   **B**

Fig. 4.52 Preparing to form an anastomosis. **A** Non-crushing bowel clamps steady the ends and prevent leakage of content. Some clamps can be locked together. **B** The ends are held together with traction sutures. If the bowel cannot be rotated, insert these not at the ends but slightly on to the back wall, so that when they are distracted they tauten the apposed back walls, leaving the anterior walls slack so that the back wall stitches can be easily inserted. (I was taught this method by Mr John Cochrane.) You may distract the anterior walls with stitches or tissue forceps to improve access to the posterior walls.

made. The traditional stitch takes in all coats (Fig. 4.53), attributed to William Halsted (1852–1922), the great American surgeon. A method that is popular at present is an extramucosal or serosubmucosal technique; all layers are included with the exception of the mucosa. A seromuscular stitch apposing and sealing the serous layers was described by the Parisian surgeon Antoine Lembert (1802–1851), to prevent leakage; it does not incorporate the submucosa and is usually considered suitable only as a second-layer stitch.

4. Use a synthetic absorbable 3/0 thread. Smooth monofilament material, having no interstices where organisms can reside, is safer in the presence of contamination but is a little stiff to tie. Multifilament thread is more supple.

5. The method of stitching depends on personal choice and on the need to control the apposition of the edges. Use continuous, interrupted simple or mattress stitches passed vertically through all coats, 3–4 mm from the edge, 3–4 mm apart. Full-thickness interrupted and spiral continuous stitches are more haemostatic than mattress stitches. In either case, carefully pick up and ligate bleeding vessels before starting the anastomotic suture.

6. The anastomotic line may lie in the sagittal or

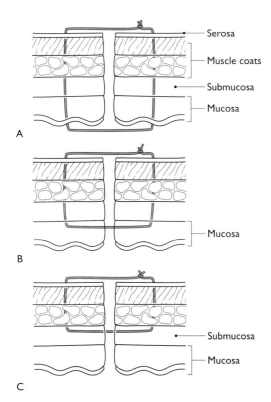

A — Serosa
— Muscle coats
— Submucosa
— Mucosa

B — Mucosa

C — Submucosa
— Mucosa

Fig. 4.53 **A** The all-coats stitch. **B** An extramucosal or serosubmucosal stitch. **C** The seromuscular or Lembert stitch.

coronal planes; it is usually easier to sew progressively from far to near when it lies in the coronal plane, progressively from dominant to non-dominant side when it lies in the sagittal plane. In each case your hand starts fully pronated and drives the curved needle through by progressively supinating (see Ch. 3, pp. 37–39).

7. Your intention must be to appose the edges perfectly, just bringing into contact the same layers of each edge. The stitches cause inflammation, producing oedema. If you have pulled the stitches too tight, they cut off the blood supply and result in delayed healing, ulceration of the mucosa or, worse, cutting out with potential leakage.

8. The methods I shall describe are applicable throughout the bowel.

9. On completion, check that the lumen is patent; carefully confirm that you can invaginate the walls from each side through the anastomotic ring.

> 🔑 **Key point**
>
> ● Check the colour of the bowel, the integrity of the blood supply and if there is a mesentery to be closed, exclude haematoma that may subsequently prejudice healing.

Mobile bowel, edge to edge, single layer, interrupted stitches

1. Insert sutures joining the anterior walls. Carefully avoid picking up the back wall. Tie the knots on the outside of the bowel.

2. When you have completed the anterior wall, turn the bowel over to bring what was the back wall to the front and insert a series of sutures to close this, completing the anastomosis (Fig. 4.54).

3. If you used stay sutures, cut these out or tie them.

4. Carefully check the mesenteric and antimesenteric edges of the bowel – the junctions of the anterior and posterior suture lines are most likely to have defects. Insert extra sutures if necessary.

5. If there is a mesentery, carefully close it with stitches, avoiding injury to, or constriction of, the vessels supplying the bowel.

Fig. 4.54 If the bowel is mobile, suture the front wall, taking care to avoid the back wall. Now turn over the bowel to bring the previous back wall to the front and close it. If the bowel has a mesentery, carefully close the defect.

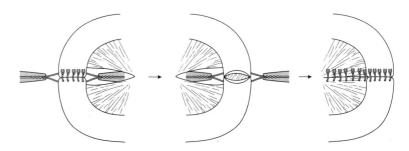

Edge to edge, single layer, continuous stitches

1. Starting on the back wall insert a stitch at one end from outside in on one side, inside out on the other side, and tie it. Clip the short end, insert the needle back through into the lumen and introduce a continuous, unlocked, spiral stitch joining the back walls as far as the other end.

2. If the line of anastomosis lies in the sagittal plane, start at the near end, complete the stitching of the back wall, continue round the far corner and close the anterior walls from far to near, to reach the starting point. If you continue the spiral stitch on to the anterior wall you will discover you have to stitch from left to right. To avoid this, at the far end, having passed the needle through to the left side, reverse the needle and pass it from within out, creating a loop on the mucosa – a single 'Connell' stitch. You can now continue to sew from right to left along the anterior wall to reach the starting point. Remove and discard the needle and tie the free end to the clamped short end.

3. If the line of anastomosis lies in the transverse (coronal) plane, start at the right end (Fig. 4.55). Insert the first stitch from without in, then from within out, tie the stitch and clamp the short end. Re-insert the needle from without in on the near side. Carry on with the over and over spiral stitches uniting the back walls from right to left. Again, at the left end, having taken the last stitch from far to near, reverse the needle to create a single Connell (mattress stitch with a loop on the mucosal aspect) stitch, coming out on the near side. You can now continue on the anterior suture line from left to right, inserting stitches from far to near. When you reach the right end, cut off the needle and tie the free end to the clamped short end.

4. Check that the anastomosis is patent.

Fixed bowel, single layer, interrupted stitches

1. This method is particularly applicable in the large bowel to anastomoses with the rectum, which lies against the sacrum and cannot be rotated. In addition, access is limited, so the anastomosis is fashioned not at the surface but in the depths.

> **Key points**
>
> - Do not unite the bowel ends under tension or they will surely distract.
> - Take particular care when inserting and tying sutures in situations that are inaccessible following completion of the procedure. This applies particularly to the posterior layer sutures in colorectal anastomoses.

2. Unite the posterior layers using carefully placed all-coats stitches, with the knots tied within the lumen. If the bowel is fixed, and subsequent access will be greatly restricted, place these stitches with the bowel ends apart, clipping but not tying them until they are all inserted. Now, keeping the sutures taut and in the correct order, slide the mobile end down to lie accurately apposed to the fixed edge of bowel and tie them (Fig. 4.56). This is the 'parachute' technique. Leave the outer ligature ends long for the present but cut the ligature ends of the remainder, leaving the knots on the interior of the bowel.

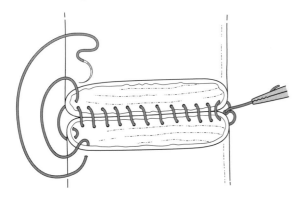

Fig. 4.55 Bowel anastomosis by continuous suture. The anastomotic line lies transversely. Start at the right side, insert an all-coats stitch and tie it. Enter the needle from without in on the near side. Unite the back walls with a spiral over-and–over stitch. At the left end insert a single Connell stitch on the near side and then continue from left to right on the anterior wall, to reach the first stitch and tie off. If you rotate the drawing 90° to the right (clockwise) it demonstrates the method when the anastomotic line lies in the sagittal plane.

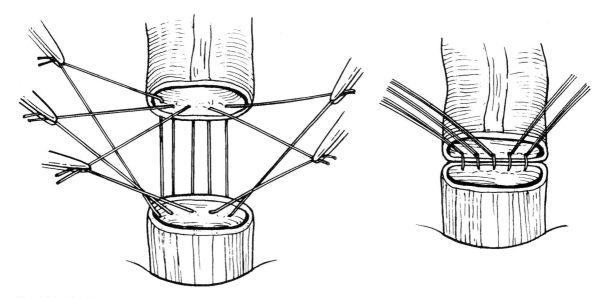

Fig. 4.56 If the bowel cannot be rotated, insert the back wall stitches, tying the knots within the lumen. In case of difficulty, leave the ends apart while you insert all the back wall stitches, slide the mobile end along the stitches and only then tie the knots. This is the 'parachute' technique.

3. Many colorectal surgeons use inverting, longitudinal (vertical) mattress sutures for the back wall (see Ch. 3, Fig. 3.66, p. 39)). These pass out through all coats at a distance from the edge, enter the other bowel end at a similar distance from the edge, then take a small bite of each of the edges before being tied within the lumen.

4. Insert interrupted inverting anterior stitches to complete the anastomosis. These may be simple or inverting longitudinal mattress stitches. Because I was taught that bowel must be sutured using all-coats stitches as a basis, I should favour these. Many colorectal surgeons employ extramucosal or even seromuscular stitches with success.

5. Because a colorectal anastomosis transmits solid faeces, it is vital to exclude defects or leaks that might disrupt the union or allow leakage with consequent infection. First, insert a finger through the anus to feel the integrity of the anastomosis. Insert a narrow-bore rigid sigmoidoscope and inspect it. Finally fill the pelvis with sterile fluid and gently inflate the rectal stump with air through the sigmoidoscope. If no bubbles appear, this suggests that the anastomosis in satisfactory.

Two-layer anastomosis

In the past the stomach and bowel were routinely and very satisfactorily sutured using two layers. The inner, all-coats stitch inverts the bowel wall. This is reinforced with an absorbable or non-absorbable outer seromuscular Lembert stitch. Although most surgeons have converted to single-layer techniques, many surgeons, adept in the two-layer technique, continue to use it and obtain good results with it.

Variations

1. Anastomoses can be made not only end to end but also end to side and side to side (Fig. 4.57). In each circumstance ensure that the holes match each other.

2. Mechanical stapling devices are frequently used for joining bowel. Some, like the circular stapler, invert the bowel and apply a double row of metal staples. Others, like some straight stapling devices, apply a double row of staples to the everted edges; most, but not all, surgeons invert the staple line with stitches. In some situations, mechanical methods are convenient. Do not assume, however, that mechanical devices can be used more rapidly or more effectively than hand sewing. They demand careful placement.

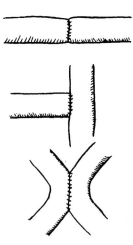

Fig. 4.57 In addition to end-to-end anastomoses, the bowel can be joined end to side and side to side.

OTHER DUCTS

1. Ureters undergo peristalsis to transmit the content but this may be impaired if the myenteric nerves or vascular supply are damaged. It is often worth cutting the ends obliquely to obviate producing an annular, constricting anastomosis.

2. Bile ducts have insufficient muscle in their walls to constrict, so they transmit contents passively. If they are injured, they often require to be united to another conduit, such as the jejunum. Bile is extremely penetrating, and leaks if the anastomosis is imperfect.

3. Anastomosis of the fallopian tubes and vas deferens in order to restore continuity following disease or previous division is usually carried out using magnification.

4. Anastomosis of small ducts is almost always performed using a single row of interrupted, all-coats sutures. The fear is that a continuous encircling suture may have a constricting effect.

> **Key point**
>
> ● Every stitch must unite the epithelial linings of the anastomosis. Fail, and a leak or stricture will follow.

5. Use fine needle and thread to produce perfect, leak-free union. However it is sutured, a straightforward end-to-end union produces a potential annular constriction ring. The postoperative oedema may block the lumen and rising pressure can then rupture the anastomosis, with subsequent leakage. To avoid this, the anastomosis can be made over a 'T-tube' or straight tube (Fig. 4.58). If necessary check the anastomosis and the 'run off,' using radio-opaque contrast medium before you withdraw a splinting tube. The leakage from the side hole will rapidly heal provided there is no distal obstruction. A double pigtailed catheter can conveniently be inserted into a repaired ureter with the upper loop in the pelvis of the ureter and the lower one in the bladder; it can be captured and extracted using a cystoscope.

6. If access is difficult, as in the depths, place the stitches while the ducts lie apart before sliding them together – the 'parachute' technique (Fig. 4.59).

7. Be willing to slit the end of a small duct so that you can join it into a similar duct that has also been slit. The slit duct can also be joined to the end or side of a wide duct (Fig. 4.60). If necessary use stay sutures to hold the ducts in apposition while you insert the stitches.

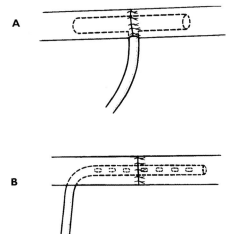

Fig. 4.58 **A** Insert a T-tube at the site of the anastomosis to splint the union. This channels the contents through the anastomosis or drains it externally. **B** The same effect is achieved by inserting a straight tube with side holes.

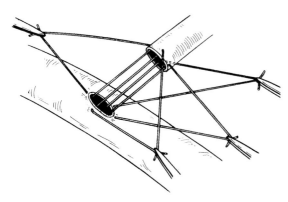

Fig. 4.59 Epithelium-to-epithelium anastomosis of small ducts is achieved by inserting the stitches while the ducts lie apart, then sliding one duct down on to the other.

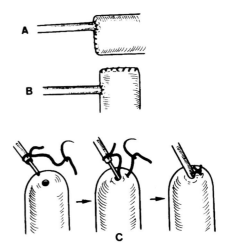

Fig. 4.61 Joining small ducts into larger ones. **A** End to end. **B** End to side. **C** Using a plastic cannula to aid union of a small duct with a large one.

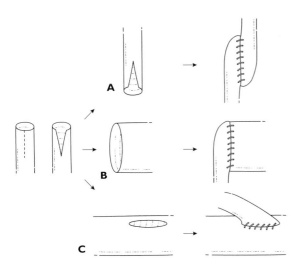

Fig. 4.60 Slit the end of a small duct to produce a wide opening. **A** Join it to another small duct, similarly split. **B** Join it to the end of a wide duct. **C** Join it into the side of a wide duct.

8. You may close the end of a large open-ended duct until it will fit the end of a small duct. Alternatively, close the end completely, joining the small duct into a freshly made opening (Fig. 4.61). Very small ducts are best cannulated with a plastic catheter, which is tied in before using it as an intro-ducer. If you leave the needled thread intact following ligation, pass the needle into the accepting hole and out nearby, so you can tie the end to the other end of the ligature to fix the duct in place. To prevent leakage, insert a purse-string suture around the anastomosis, gently push in the duct and tie the purse-string suture, producing an 'inkwell' effect.

BOWEL TRANSFER

Bowel, which has a rich blood supply, can be transferred to a different site, but must retain or regain a blood supply to survive. A segment of bowel can be transferred elsewhere, while preserving its blood supply, by opening out the arching blood vessels that run in its mesentery to supply it from one end. The other end can be extended (Fig. 4.62). This was first described by the brilliant Swiss surgeon César Roux (1851–1934) in 1908. If it is necessary to transfer the segment at a distance, the blood vessels can be divided and reimplanted into vessels near the recipient site (Fig. 4.63). This demands highly skilled microvascular surgery (see Ch. 5).

SPHINCTERS

● Localized segments of specially controlled circular muscle meters and regulates the rate and direction of flow. These are sphincters (G

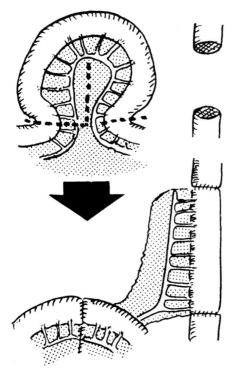

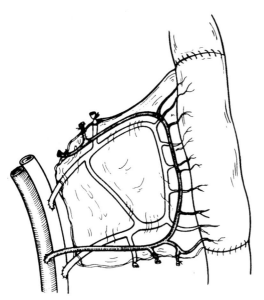

Fig. 4.62 Transferring bowel while retaining its blood supply. At the top, the dotted line shows the line of section. Open the loop out and join it into place as shown in the lower diagram.

Fig. 4.63 Bowel removed from one site has its blood vessels joined into those at the new site. As a rule, two veins are anastomosed for each artery.

sphingein = to bind tightly). They may or may not be anatomically obvious.

- Inadvertent damage to the muscle or nerve supply may be irrevocable.
- Dilatation or overstretching often puts the sphincter out of action. It can be achieved in a similar manner to correcting a stricture, by passing graded bougies or balloon dilatation. If the sphincter is overstretched the muscle is disrupted and may never recover. If the muscle is torn the resulting fibrosis may produce stenosis.

Myotomy

1. Divide a clearly defined circular muscle forming a sphincter, using a longitudinal incision while leaving the lining intact (Fig. 4.64). Perform this when the sphincter is overdeveloped, or fails to relax, so that the contents cannot pass.

2. In *infantile hypertrophic pyloric stenosis* the operation is called pyloromyotomy and may be performed under local or general anaesthesia. Lift out the pylorus with fingers or tissue forceps. Hold it steady while carefully incising the thickened muscle, leaving the mucosa intact and bulging into the gap. Gently lift remaining fibres, using a hook or fine non-toothed forceps, and cut them. Pick up each side of the cut edge, using gauze swabs to improve your grip, and gently separate the edges, or use round-nosed forceps to lever the edges apart. Sometimes you can

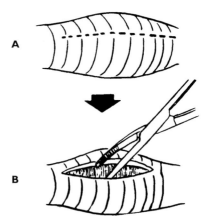

Fig. 4.64 Myotomy. Divide the sphincter **(A)** along the dotted line. Split the edges apart **(B)** to ensure that the circular muscle is totally divided.

collect a little air into the segment to bulge the mucosa and exclude or identify any leak. If there is a break in the mucosa, carefully suture it, perhaps drawing over it a tag of tissue such as omentum.

3. Myotomy of the lower oesophageal sphincter overcomes the condition of achalasia (G *a* = not + *chalaein* = to relax) of the cardia of the stomach. Like pyloromyotomy, it is intended that the underlying mucosa remains intact. The operation was described by Ernst Heller of Leipzig in 1913.

Sphincterotomy

1. Divide the whole thickness, including the duct lining, when the sphincter controls the termination of a spouted duct (Fig. 4.65). The ampulla of Abraham Vater (1684–1751, of Wittemberg in Germany), usually accepts both the common bile and pancreatic ducts. Through an opening in the duodenum, insinuate one blade of a pair of scissors into the spout and cut through with the other blade. Alternatively pass in a grooved probe and cut down into the groove with a scalpel. This type of sphincterotomy is now usually performed through a fibreoptic endoscope, using a diathermy wire.

2. *Anal fissure* can be successfully treated by dividing the lower internal sphincter. The fissure nearly always lies in the midline posteriorly but carry out the sphincterotomy on the lateral wall. Insert a proctoscope with an open slot that reveals the lateral anal wall. Make a small circumferential incision at the anal margin. Through this insert closed blunt-ended scissors beneath the mucosa and gently open them to separate the mucosa and lower internal sphincter. Withdraw the scissors, close them and again insert them, this time deep to the lower internal sphincter, and open them to separate it from the external sphincter. Remove the scissors and introduce a straight haemostat, one blade superficial to, one blade deep to the internal sphincter, clamp it, open it and withdraw it. With the scissors now cut vertically through the crushed sphincter to the upper level of the fissure.

Sphincteroplasty

If you perform sphincterotomy, the raw edges may rejoin. However, if you join the inner and outer epithelia with sutures, the opening will remain patulous (Fig. 4.66). When a sphincter surrounds a duct in continuity, such as the pylorus, incise longitudinally through it, widely separate the walls and suture the defect as a transverse suture line. At the pylorus this manoeuvre is referred to as a **pyloroplasty**. It is a method of overcoming stenosis that results from chronic peptic ulcer in the proximal duodenum, with consequent scar contracture.

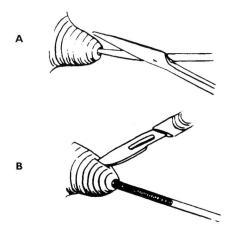

Fig. 4.65 Sphincterotomy. **A** Introduce one blade of the scissors into the mouth of the duct to cut through the encircling sphincter. **B** Introduce a grooved probe into the duct and cut down on to it with a scalpel.

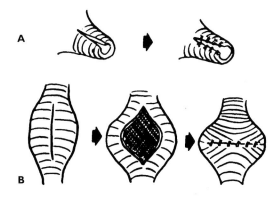

Fig. 4.66 Sphincteroplasty. **A** Divide a terminal sphincter and stitch the inner and outer linings together. **B** Divide the sphincter longitudinally, widely separate the edges and sew up the defect as a transverse suture line.

Sphincter repair

A sphincter may need to be cut deliberately. The sphincteric opening of the vagina may be deliberately divided during delivery in the operation of episiotomy (G *epision* = pubes, pudenda + *temnien* = to cut) to avoid an uncontrolled tear. This can be sewn up successfully in most cases. Repair of old sphincteric defects or tears is usually less successful; it is usually helpful to excise the edges of the old, scarred sphincter and carry out a fresh repair (Fig. 4.67)

Sphincter reversal

Some sphincters act unidirectionally, rather like valves. Indeed, as a rule, though not always, the direction of peristaltic action in the bowel is unidirectional so that it acts like a one-way valve. In order to slow down the passage in the hope of allowing more time for absorption following massive bowel resection, it is possible to take out a segment, still attached by its blood and nerve supply, reverse it, and restore it into continuity (Fig. 4.68).

ACQUIRED CHANNELS AND CAVITIES

These are varied in origin, including developmental, traumatic, infective, resulting from the presence of foreign material, and neoplastic.

SINUS

1. The lining of the channel may be granulation tissue but it may become epithelialized. In some cases removing the cause may suffice, in others the whole track needs to be excised.

2. The most common sinus (L = something hollowed out, a bay) you will see is a wound sinus. A superficial stitch often acts as a foreign body, especially if it has a long, stiff cut end lying beneath the skin, which eventually protrudes. In some cases the wound sinus may be caused by a piece of necrotic tissue or missed foreign material. Initially, try to insert fine 'mosquito' artery forceps, gently open the blades and attempt to capture the stitch or other cause

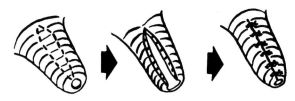

Fig. 4.67 Sphincter repair. Excise the edges to expose the fresh, raw ends of the sphincter before suturing them together.

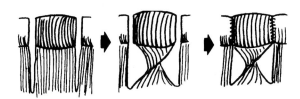

Fig. 4.68 Sphincter reversal. Take out of continuity the sphincteric segment, still attached to its blood supply, reverse it and restore it into continuity.

and remove it. If this fails, be willing to explore the sinus under local anaesthesia, enlarging the opening until you can see the cause and remove it.

3. A classical condition is pilonidal sinus (L *pilum* = hair + *nidus* = nest). Hair driven beneath the skin over the coccyx forms a source of chronic irritation and often infection. It has an external opening. In the past it was often widely excised as though it was a malignancy. It is now usually treated successfully by opening up the channel to the surface, scrupulously removing all the hairs and keeping the mouth widely open while the cavity fills up from the depths (Fig. 4.69) to obliterate itself.

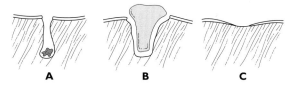

Fig. 4.69 Sinus. **A** A sinus with foreign material, diseased tissue, or hair within a pilonidal sinus. **B** The irritant cause of chronicity has been removed, the opening has been widened and the cavity packed so that it fills the base. **C** The base has filled with granulation tissue, which contracts while epithelium grows in to heal over.

FISTULA

1. The term (L = pipe) is used in medicine to signify a pipe open at both ends on to an epithelial surface. In some cases, removing the cause may succeed but if the track becomes completely epithelialized it will never close spontaneously. If there is infection, foreign material, neoplasia and a high rate of flow through the track it is unlikely to heal, especially if the discharge is irritant. This applies if a fistula develops from, for example, the biliary system or the bowel. The fistula will never heal if there is distal obstruction and the fistulous track is acting as a safety channel.

2. In some circumstances, as when a fistulous tract relieves an impassable or unresectable obstruction, the fistula is beneficial. If a serious leakage occurs into a large compartment such as the peritoneal cavity, containment as a result of the development of a fistulous track spares the patient possible generalized peritonitis.

3. A fistula-in-ano results from inflammation in or near the (usually) lower bowel, often with infection and abscess formation that sometimes 'points' towards the perianal skin so that a track develops between the bowel and skin. A probe can usually be passed from the external orifice through the track into the bowel. If the track is now laid open (Fig. 4.70) and subsequently kept open until new tissue has filled the defect it may heal. This cannot always be achieved if the internal opening is high, because it entails dividing too much of the anal sphincter muscles that maintain anal continence.

STOMA

1. The term (G = mouth) applies to a natural or artificial mouth between an internal duct and another duct, another part of the same channel, or the exterior. For example, the mouth is a natural stoma; union of the stomach and intestine is a gastroenterostomy (G *enteron* = L *intestine*, from *intus* = within); the exteriorization of the colon to the skin is a colostomy.

2. Provided the lining of the two surfaces fuse, the stoma is stable. If fusion does not occur, or if the epithelium is destroyed, fibrosis develops and as this matures it contracts so that the stoma constricts. For this reason, if you wish to form a permanent stoma, as when joining intestine at an anastomosis, joining ducts or uniting a duct into the bowel, ensure that the epithelium and mucosa are sutured into perfect contact (Fig. 4.71). In the past, surgeons often brought bowel to the surface without uniting the mucosa to skin. As a result a frequently performed operation was 'refashioning of colostomy'.

CYSTS

1. Some cysts (G *kystis* = bladder, bag or pouch) are developmental, such as a branchial cyst (G *branchion* = gill). If an epithelium such as skin is detached and buried, it grows until it meets other cells of the same tissue, resulting in an *implantation cyst*. If the emptying channel of a secretory gland is blocked, the gland may distend and become cystic. Some diseases, including neoplasms result in cyst formation.

2. One method of dealing with a cyst is to excise

Fig. 4.70 Fistula. **A** Diagram of an anal fistulous track communicating between the anal canal and the perianal skin. **B** A malleable probe has been passed through the track and the intervening tissue has been divided (cross-hatched portion), exposing the track in the bottom of the cleft you have created (**C**) when seen from the perineal aspect. **D** As a result of the packing and other measures to prevent the edges from bridging over, the cleft is shallow, smaller, and will shortly heal.

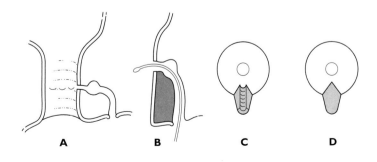

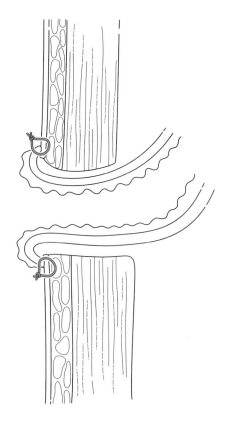

local anaesthesia; prefer to use a fairly large volume of dilute anaesthetic injected not into but around the cyst. This separates the capsule from the surrounding tissue, greatly facilitating the subsequent sharp dissection and reducing bleeding. If you fail to excise all the secretory lining of a cystic gland, it is liable to reform.

3. The most common cyst with which you will have to deal is a sebaceous cyst (see Ch. 6, p. 108).

4. A retention cyst near a surface can often be decapitated by removing the overlying tissue. The epithelium of the surface rapidly fuses with the lining of the cyst (Fig. 4.72). Salivary cysts within the mouth are amenable to this treatment.

5. Occasionally, a cavity such as a cyst can be treated by introducing a tube attached to a suction device, which draws the walls together so that it collapses and shrivels.

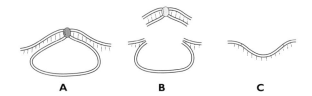

Fig. 4.71 External stoma. Diagram through a stoma in which the end of the bowel has been brought to the surface through a hole made in the abdominal wall. The end of the bowel wall has been everted so that the mucosa can be stitched directly to the skin.

it without opening it, avoiding spilling the contents. This applies to ovarian, branchial and epididymal (G *epi* = upon + *didymos* = twin; it was an old term for both testes and ovaries) cysts. A retention cyst such as a sebaceous cyst can usually be excised under

Fig. 4.72 De-roofing a cyst. **A** A retention cyst: the secretions cannot escape because the mouth of the glandular cyst is stenosed. **B** The overlying epithelium and the roof of the cyst have been removed. **C** The lining of the cyst and the epithelium have fused at the edges and the surface gradually becomes uniform.

ABSCESSES

See Chapter 12.

5

Handling blood vessels

with George Hamilton

Percutaneous puncture
Percutaneous cannulation
Percutaneous catheterization
Sutures
Expose and control (see Ch. 10)
Incision
Veins – direct procedures
Varicose veins
Arterial replacement with vein
Arteries – direct procedures
Incision and closure
Direct catheterization
Embolectomy
Vein patch
Anastomosis
Microvascular surgery

- Transmission of blood is by vis a tergo (L *vis* = force, compulsion + *a tergo* = from behind, from *tergum* = the back). Blood vessels do not undergo peristalsis.
- The size of the channel does not automatically respond to the volume of fluid passing through it – arteries or veins may constrict as a result of smooth muscle contraction at a time when there is an increased demand for vascular transport.
- The need to maintain a continuous normal endothelial surface has unique surgical implications. Blood tends to clot on denuded areas, reducing the lumen or completely obstructing it. Platelets adhere to damaged intact intima, also promoting blood clots.
- Vein walls are thinner than arteries, since the pressure of blood is normally lower than that in the arteries. Many veins are valved so that they

transmit blood in only one direction. Because the blood flow is usually slower than in arteries, there is an increased tendency for clotting to occur if the endothelium is damaged, if there is stagnation or if there is a clotting diathesis (G = a predisposition, from *diatithenai* = to dispose).

- Arteries (G *arteria* = windpipe – after death the arteries are empty and so were thought to transmit air) have thicker walls than veins. Diseased arteries may be rigid and stenosed and the intima easily separates from the media, because of deposition of subintimal fatty atheroma (G *athara* = porridge + *-oma* = tumour or swelling; Fig. 5.1).
- For local anticoagulation in arterial surgery, use 500 ml isotonic saline containing 5000 international units (IU) heparin to flush and instil locally.

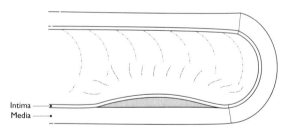

Fig. 5.1 Subintimal deposition of atheroma separating endothelium from the media.

PERCUTANEOUS PUNCTURE

Veins

1. Veins are most easily entered when they are distended. They constrict in hypovolaemia, as a result of cold and as a result of local trauma. Veins

> ### Key point
>
> - Your skill in gaining access to veins is frequently called on, often in emergency circumstances with collapsed, deeply placed veins. Do not attempt venepuncture until you have confidently identified the anatomy. Repeated failure erodes your confidence.

distend if they are warm, placed dependently or mildly congested; this last can often be achieved by simple finger pressure restricting venous return. In the limbs, place a cuff that obstructs venous return but not arterial inflow, and the effect can be augmented if the subject performs repeated muscle contractions of the part. Use a warm hot water bottle or hair dryer to encourage local venous filling.

2. Do not overcongest veins, especially in elderly people, or they rupture spontaneously or when punctured.

3. Ensure that the lighting is adequate – tangential lighting may be helpful by producing shadowing of the dilated vein. Be prepared to shave overlying hair to improve the view. A deeply sited vein can often be identified if you place one finger over the likely site while gently tapping it proximally or peripherally; your 'watching' finger detects the thrill. Some veins can be entered because their anatomical position, the site of puncture, direction and depth of needle insertion have been well described, such as the subclavian and femoral veins. In case of doubt, confirm the presence of the vein using a Doppler ultrasound detector.

4. If you must insert a large needle, or carry out a subsequent manoeuvre, and especially if the patient is apprehensive, first inject a small volume of local anaesthetic through a fine needle very superficially in the skin; after allowing a few minutes to allow it to take effect, insert the needle through the bleb. To aid insertion of a large needle or one carrying an external cannula, first make a small incision with a pointed scalpel. The needle then slides easily through the superficial tissues and the 'feel' is not lost, as it is when the needle is tightly gripped by skin.

5. Elderly patients often have veins that are thick-

walled, slippery and difficult to fix while puncturing them. Apply a finger or thumb just beside the vein and draw it distally to slightly stretch the vessel (Fig. 5.2). If you press too close to the vein or apply too strong traction, you will collapse it and your finger obstructs the line of needle insertion. When the site of insertion lies just proximal to a joint, exert gentle traction by flexing the joint (Fig. 5.3); the finger placed beside the vein no longer threatens to obstruct the path of the needle.

6. Insert the needle, with the bevel uppermost, almost vertically through the skin, since the longer its track within the skin the more uncomfortable the prick. Now direct it so that it lies close to, and parallel to, the vein. Angle the tip so that it 'squashes' gently into the vein to enter the lumen (Fig. 5.4). Check this by gently aspirating blood into the syringe, then advance the needle within the vein but avoid introducing the whole needle; if it breaks

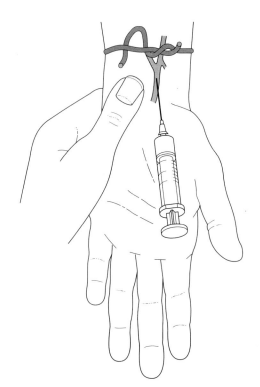

Fig. 5.2 Venepuncture. Your left thumb fixes the vein just to one side to allow the needle to align with the vein. Your thumb draws down the skin and vein to fix but not compress the vein. Insert the needle with the bevel uppermost.

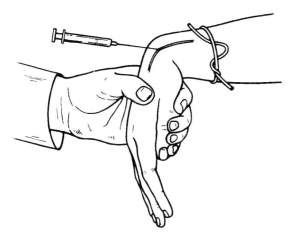

Fig. 5.3 Place your thumb near the vein distally and flex the wrist so that your hand does not impinge on the alignment of the needle.

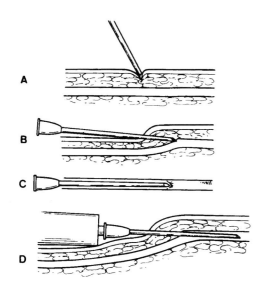

Fig. 5.4 **A** Pierce the skin almost vertically. **B** Align the needle almost parallel to the vein and prepare to 'squash' it into the vein. Notice that the bevel is uppermost. **C** View from above shows the needle in the line of the vein, exactly over it. **D** The needle enters the vein, accurately lined up with it.

at the Luer connection the shaft cannot be grasped and withdrawn.

7. When attempting to puncture thick-walled, slippery veins, or those that cannot be fully congested because they are fragile, look for a junction where the vein is tethered by the tributaries (Fig. 5.5).

> ### 🔑 Key point
>
> - Do not withdraw the needle until you have removed the congesting cuff.

8. Apply gentle pressure through a sterile swab over the puncture site while you extract the needle and maintain the pressure for 3 minutes, timed by the clock.

9. Do not rely on needles for long-term infusion into veins. Needles soon pull out, or penetrate the vein wall allowing the fluid to 'tissue'.

10. When you require repeated access, as for haemodialysis in patients with chronic renal failure, you will need to create an arteriovenous fistula anastomosing the radial artery to the cephalic vein. The increased pressure in the vein distends it and it can be used repeatedly.

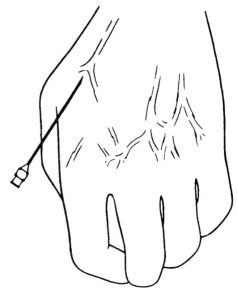

Fig. 5.5 The needle is about to enter a superficial vein at the junction of tributaries where the draining vessel is relatively fixed.

Arteries

1. Arteries are often mobile and if they are thick-walled in elderly or hypertensive people they may slip from under a needle or be difficult to puncture.

2. Raise a bleb of local anaesthetic in the skin at

the site of puncture and infiltrate the tissues around the artery. Make a small stab through the skin with a pointed scalpel blade. This important step allows you to slide the needle easily down to the vessel, so that you can 'feel' the entry into it; only now is it gripped as you advance it.

3. Fix the artery if possible by pressing it against a firm base (Fig. 5.6).

4. Insert the needle with the bevel uppermost until it lies on the artery, then enter the artery at an angle, when small spurts of blood enter the syringe. The pressure required to puncture a thick-walled artery may collapse it, so make short jerky movements.

5. In case of difficulty it may be less damaging to transfix the artery cleanly and then slowly withdraw the needle until blood spurts into the syringe, rather than repeatedly stabbing into the thick wall (Fig. 5.7).

6. Needles are not suitable for prolonged retention in an artery since they damage the endothelium and may penetrate the vessel wall or become dislodged, allowing leakage to occur.

7. When you withdraw the needle have a sterile pad available to press on the puncture site; maintain

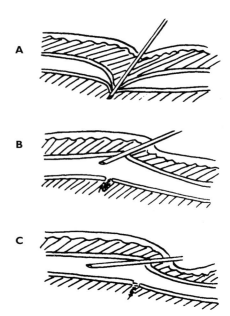

Fig. 5.7 Percutaneous arterial puncture. Rather than make repeated damaging attempts, (**A**) transfix the artery, gradually withdraw the needle (**B**) until blood spurts into the syringe, then (**C**) advance the needle within the lumen of the artery.

this for at least 5 minutes timed by the clock, depending on the patient's clotting status.

PERCUTANEOUS CANNULATION

Cannula (L = reed) suggests a stiff tube. Most modern vascular cannulas are commercially produced plastic sheaths fitted closely on needles, the distal part of the cannula being chamfered smoothly on to the shank of the needle (Fig. 5.8). A disadvantage of this cannula is that it cannot be longer than the needle. However, it has the advantage over a needle in that the plastic cannula is unlikely to damage or perforate the vessel wall from within. Moreover, it provides an adequate channel for the passage of a variety of catheters, guide wires and other instruments.

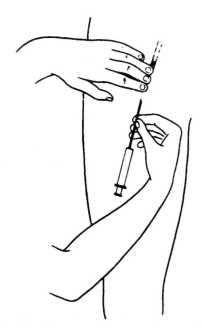

Fig. 5.6 Percutaneous puncture of an artery. Locate and fix it with your non-dominant hand.

> 🔑 **Key point**
>
> • Never reintroduce a partially or completely withdrawn needle into the cannula. The needle may penetrate the plastic cannula wall, detach it and create a foreign body embolus.

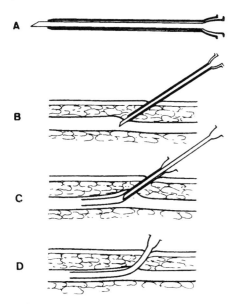

Fig. 5.8   A The closely fitting cannula is smoothly chamfered distally on to the needle. **B** The needle enters the vessel; then hold it steady. **C** Advance the cannula over the needle. **D** Withdraw the needle, leaving the cannula in place.

Veins

1. To introduce the cannula, proceed as for percutaneous puncture. First, raise a bleb of local anaesthetic, wait 5 minutes then create a small punctured incision to accommodate the needle and cannula. When you enter the vein, gently advance it against the increasing resistance as the tip of the cannula smoothly expands the hole to enter the lumen. Be careful to maintain the tip of the needle central within the vein, to avoid damaging or perforating the wall.

2. When you are confident that the cannula has entered the vein, hold the needle still while gently advancing the cannula. Now withdraw the needle after preparing to connect or control the cannula.

3. If you are in doubt about the correct siting of the cannula, connect a syringe and confirm that blood can be aspirated.

Arteries

> **Key point**
>
> - Do not start until you are confident that you have identified the artery.

1. Proceed initially as for percutaneous venous cannulation. When you enter the artery, gently advance the cannula against the increasing resistance as its tip smoothly expands the hole to enter the lumen.

2. Be careful to maintain the tip of the needle central within the artery, to avoid damaging or perforating the wall.

3. Watch carefully for incipient leakage producing a haematoma while you are trying to insert the needle and cannula. Withdraw the cannula and compress the site for 5 minutes by the clock. Move to a fresh site.

4. When you are confident that the cannula has entered the artery, gently advance it while holding the needle still. Now withdraw the needle after preparing to connect or control the cannula.

5. Confirm that blood spurts into the syringe.

6. Carefully and gently compress the entry site for 5 minutes times by the clock.

PERCUTANEOUS CATHETERIZATION

- Hippocrates used the term catheter (G *kata* = down + *hienai* = to send) for an instrument for emptying the bladder. Like cannulas, they were also stiff tubes until the French surgeon Auguste Nélaton in 1860 invented the rubber catheter. Intravenous catheters are made of plastic tubing.
- Catheters may be inserted into veins or arteries.
- They can be passed through needles or cannulas, provided their external diameter is less than the internal diameter of the needle or cannula (Fig. 5.9). When the needle is withdrawn it cannot be removed from the catheter, if this has an external Luer connection, unless the needle is of a special type that can be split and opened longitudinally.

1. In the *Seldinger technique* developed by the American radiologist in 1953, a flexible guide wire can be inserted through a needle or a cannula. Leave the guide wire within the vessel and withdraw the needle or cannula. Now thread a catheter over the guide-wire (Fig. 5.10). If necessary, first pass hollow dilators over the guide wire and finally pass a large-bore, thin-walled cannula through which a large-bore catheter can be inserted (Fig. 5.11).

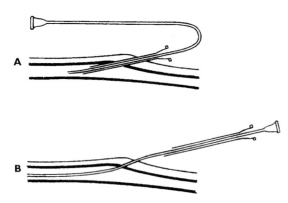

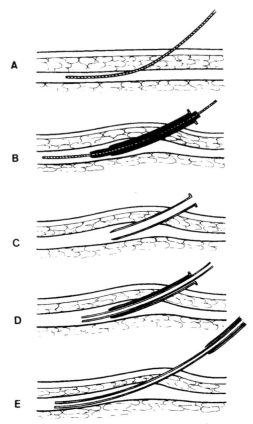

Fig. 5.9 Inserting a blunt catheter percutaneously using a sharp needle as a pilot. **A** shows a catheter passed through the lumen of the needle. **B** shows the needle withdrawn.

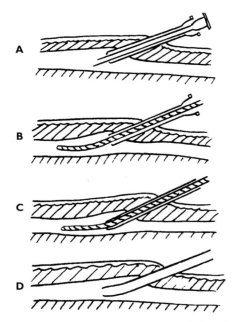

Fig. 5.10 Seldinger's guide wire technique. **A** Cannulate the vessel. **B** Withdraw the needle and replace it with the guide wire. **C** Withdraw the cannula and replace it with the plastic catheter. **D** Remove the guide wire.

Fig. 5.11 **A** The Seldinger wire has been passed into the vessel. **B** Pass the dilator, carrying the insertion cannula, into the vessel, over the guide wire. **C** Withdraw the guide wire and dilator, leaving the cannula in place. **D** Pass the catheter through the cannula into the vessel. **E** Withdraw the cannula.

🔑 Key point

- Those who perform these procedures have acquired a skill that is increasingly exploited – the manipulation of implements viewed on monitor screens, not seen directly. Familiarize yourself with the techniques.

2. Catheters can be inserted for long distances and guided (Fig. 5.12) to specific points for many purposes, including collection of specimens, delivery of substances, pressure measurements, radiological diagnosis, embolization of vessels, and insertion of balloons for dilating stenosed segments and expandable stents to maintain the lumen.

SUTURES

- Monofilament polyethylene or polyester-coated braided material are both non-absorbable, as is polytetrafluoroethylene, which is used when suturing grafts made of that material. Sutures are mounted on curved, round-bodied, eyeless

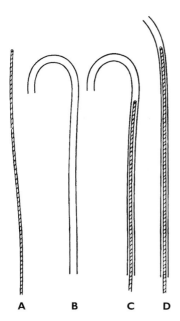

Fig. 5.12 **A** The straight guide wire alongside **(B)** the preformed curve-tipped catheter. **C** A catheter with a guide wire inserted through the straight portion of the catheter. **D** The straight guide wire is pushed into the preformed curved portion of the catheter, partially straightening it.

needles. For the aorta size 3/0 is used, with diminishing sizes as small as 8/0 for small arteries and veins. The material can be supplied with an attached needle at each end – 'double needled'.

- If the smooth surface of extruded, synthetic suture material is damaged, it is seriously weakened. Monofilament material is at greatest risk because a single break in the surface puts the whole thread at risk.

 Key point

- Do not grasp a suture with metal instruments except in segments that will be discarded, or drag it over hard, rough surfaces, or jerkily snatch it; you will reduce its strength by up to 50%.

1. Insert sutures, whenever possible, from within out. Especially when suturing diseased arteries, there is a danger that a needle passed from without in (Fig. 5.13), will separate the intima from the media. Blood

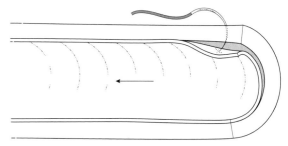

Fig. 5.13 Creation of a dissection. The arrow indicates the direction of blood flow.

can then insinuate itself beneath the endothelium, diverting the flow away from the lumen and causing progressive endothelial stripping – a dissecting aneurysm. The danger is greatest when the intima is lifted on the peripheral side of a break in continuity. For this reason, when suturing a transverse defect in an artery, start from the outside in on the upstream side, and from the inside out on the downstream side.

2. Carefully follow the curve of the needle by rotating your needle holder; if you do not you may tear out the needle or thread, or enlarge the hole, so creating a point of leakage.

3. Use non-toothed dissecting forceps held in your non-dominant hand to assist you when inserting sutures. Avoid gripping the vessel – and especially avoid grasping the endothelium. Use the forceps for counterpressure when inserting the needle; it is often convenient to allow the blades to separate slightly while you drive the needle through the vessel wall to emerge between them (Fig. 5.14).

5. Stitches may be:

a. continuous: unlocked stitches are the standard method of suturing. Since they form a spiral around the circumference of an artery, each distending pulsation of the vessel tightens the spiral. Recovery of blood pressure following operation with arterial distension similarly tightens the spiral stitches, reducing the likelihood of leakage (Fig. 5.15A).

b. interrupted: single stitches are appropriate for small vessels and in paediatric surgery because they do not restrict increase in vessel circumference as growth proceeds (Fig. 5.15B). However, because stitch separation is increased when the vessel distends, there is an increased risk of bleeding if the

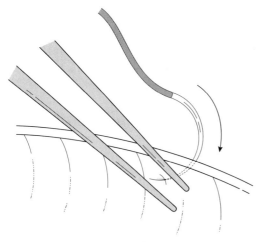

Fig. 5.14 Use slightly open dissecting forceps for counter-pressure as you drive the needle through the vessel wall, not as graspers.

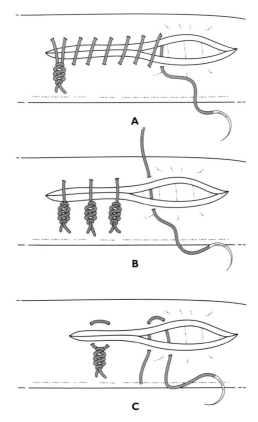

Fig. 5.15 **A** A single continuous spiral stitch. **B** Simple interrupted stitches. **C** An everting mattress stitch brings together the endothelium from each side; it may be used to initiate eversion and the line can then often be continued using simple stitches

stitches are not correctly placed, correctly tightened and tied.

c. mattress: it is not usually necessary to insert all everting mattress sutures (Fig. 5.15C) but occasionally it is valuable to start with a single one in order to initiate eversion. Mattress sutures tend to narrow the lumen. They are sometimes valuable when suturing diseased arteries, to reduce the danger of single stitches cutting out. They may also be valuable to start an anastomosis from the inside of the back wall of a fixed artery that cannot be rotated, if the walls have a tendency to invert.

7. It is usually easier to insert sutures on a curved needle mounted in a needle holder from far to near or from your dominant to non-dominant side. You insert the needle with your hand fully pronated, progressively supinating it to drive the needle through to emerge near you, or to your non-dominant side. Follow the curve of the needle. If you merely push it through, you will produce a large stitch hole, resulting in bleeding. Until you are skilled, be willing to move to the other side of the operating table in order to suture in a comfortable, practised manner.

8. When inserting stitches and drawing them to the correct tension to seal the vessel – and you must assiduously watch your masters and learn the correct tension – do not let them loosen. Pass the emerging thread to your assistant to hold without changing the tension. Repeated slackening and retightening the thread exerts a sawing effect on the vessel wall, with a tendency to cut out. It also damages the thread surface, weakening it.

> **Key point**
>
> • Every stitch must pick up the endothelium. For success, every stitch must be inserted correctly, tightened correctly and tied correctly. Do not be satisfied with 99% perfection. In order to bring the endothelium on each side of an incision or anastomosis into apposition, the edges need to be everted (Fig. 5.16).

8. Knots are potential causes of failure if they are improperly tied, either because insufficient half-

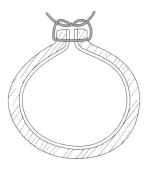

Fig. 5.16 The vessel edges must be everted in order to maintain contact between the endothelium on each side.

hitches have been used or because the material has been damaged by rough tightening. The more knots, the more potential sites of failure.

 Key point

- Monofilament synthetic material has 'memory' and a relatively friction-free surface. It is also relatively inflexible; even though you form each hitch perfectly, it is valueless unless you tighten every hitch evenly and securely. Tie as many as seven or eight correctly formed and fully tightened half-hitches, each successive one forming a reef-knot with the previous one. Leave the ends long. Of course, all knots must be on the external surface.

EXPOSE AND CONTROL (SEE CH. 10)

1. Revise the anatomy beforehand but remember that blood vessels do not always follow the usual path. Disease processes may distort and weaken vessels and surrounding tissue. Blood vessels and nerves frequently run together within a sheath. In exposing individual blood vessels, avoid damaging other structures.

2. On many occasions, veins are exposed for cosmetic reasons. Never fail to mark the intended site of incision beforehand. Place the incision to produce the best possible postoperative appearance

compatible with safe exposure, preferably parallel to the skin tension lines.

3. Gently open round-nosed haemostatic forceps on each side to expose first one side and then the other, to reveal any deeply placed branches or tributaries (Fig. 5.17).

4. Pass around the vessel proximal and distal tapes, untied ligatures or Silastic® tubing (Fig. 5.18); they may, depending on the size of the vessel, be merely

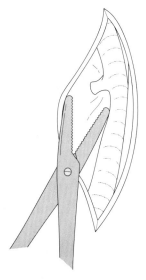

Fig. 5.17 Gently open round-nosed forceps at right angles to the artery to displace it and ensure that there is no deep tributary at risk of damage.

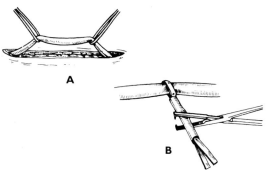

Fig. 5.18 **A** Encircle the vessel proximal and distal to the site of the procedure so that you can exert traction to tighten the tubing and occlude the lumen. **B** A tape encircles the vessel. The ends are passed through rubber tubing. If the tape ends are pulled tighter and forceps clamped across the tube, the vessel is occluded.

drawn upon to angle and occlude the vessel, or made to encircle it so that it can be constricted. Alternatively, control the vessel by applying non-damaging clamps or, for very small vessels, 'bulldog' clips (Fig. 5.19). In this way you can occlude and isolate a segment.

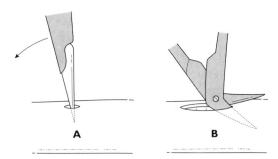

Fig. 5.20 **A** Start the incision with a pointed scalpel. **B** Extend the incision with Potts scissors.

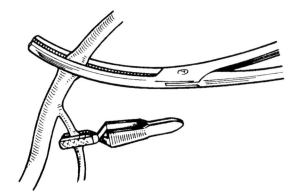

Fig. 5.19 Control of blood vessels. The larger vessel is controlled by an arterial clamp, the smaller by a spring 'bulldog' clip.

vessels are closed, clot usually forms along the suture line. The lumen is less impinged upon by a longitudinal suture line than it is by a circumferential suture line at one point (Fig. 5.21).

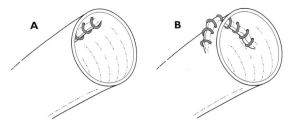

Fig. 5.21 Any clot forming on the longitudinal suture line in **A** is unlikely to cause serious obstruction but clot forming on the circumferential suture line in **B** causes marked narrowing.

INCISION

1. Avoid damaging the intima when incising veins and arteries. This may occur if you make a rough incision that penetrates to or through the back wall.

2. Diseased arteries may have loose plaques, which can be dislodged; as far as possible ensure that you make the incision in a healthy segment. The scalpel blade may also dislodge the intimal coat, separating it from the media, potentially starting a dissection.

3. Having entered the vessel, enlarge the incision using Potts scissors, ensuring that the deep blade does not damage the posterior wall (Fig. 5.20). Cut cleanly without removing and reintroducing the internal scissors blade, to avoid producing a ragged incision.

4. Because veins are thin-walled they usually accommodate to longitudinal or transverse incision. Large and medium-sized arteries may be opened transversely or longitudinally but smaller arteries are usually best opened longitudinally. When the

VEINS – DIRECT PROCEDURES

- Access to veins is a valuable means of obtaining venous blood for diagnostic purposes.
- Veins make valuable substitutes for arteries that are stenosed or blocked.
- The most common venous disease you will encounter is varicose veins, which are lengthened, dilated and with incompetent valves.

1. Before inserting a catheter that will fill the lumen and remain, place two tapes or ligatures, one above, one below the site of insertion. Make a longitudinal or transverse incision in a large vein. Insert the tip of the catheter (Fig. 5.22) and relax the proximal

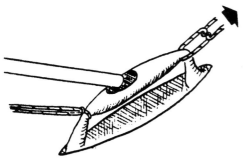

Fig. 5.22 The vein has been tied off behind the catheter. Apply traction with the ligature thread. The other ligature is left untied until you have introduced the catheter beyond it. Then tie the ligature around the vein and contained catheter to retain it.

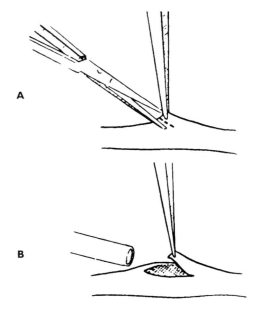

Fig. 5.24 **A** shows the vein being opened obliquely to produce a 'V' flap. In **B** the flap is raised so that the catheter can be inserted under it.

controlling ligature to allow the catheter to pass through. Tie the second ligature around the vein and catheter to retain it.

2. To introduce a small catheter into a large vein without occluding the lumen, first insert a small purse-string suture, with a formed but not tightened half-hitch, around the site of insertion. Control the vein using proximal and distal tapes, loops or non-damaging clamps. Carefully make a small stab into the vein and insert the catheter (Fig. 5.23). Fully advance it by partially releasing the appropriate occlusion device. Tighten and tie the purse string and cautiously relax the occlusion, ensuring that there is no leakage.

3. Incise small veins by lifting a small portion of the wall and cutting obliquely with scissors to raise a 'V' flap. Hold this up while slipping the fine

catheter underneath it and into the lumen (Fig. 5.24).

4. To insert a needle into an exposed very fine vein, use the ligatures on each side of the point of insertion to hold the vessel steady. It is sometimes an advantage to hold the needle in a gently closed needle holder or haemostatic forceps for better control (Fig. 5.25).

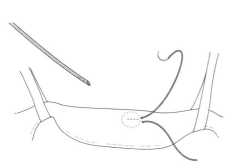

Fig. 5.23 A purse-string suture has been inserted into the vein and the straight dotted line within this indicates the site of a stab incision to accept the catheter.

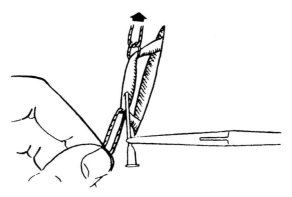

Fig. 5.25 Cannulating a very fine vessel with a needle held in a needle holder or a haemostatic forceps.

> ### Key points
>
> - Do not allow air to enter large central veins for fear of causing air embolus to the heart, consequent frothing and circulatory failure.
> - When tying off tributaries of main veins, take great care not to narrow the main vein by applying the ligature too closely. Conversely, do not leave a cul de sac, which encourages turbulence, stagnation and consequent thrombosis (Fig. 5.26).

VARICOSE VEINS

These can be treated surgically in a number of ways.

Local ties

Local ties are suitable for small, cosmetically important varicosities as an alternative to injection therapy. The procedure can be performed at the time of vein stripping.

1. If few ties are required you may use local anaesthesia. Raise a small bleb using a fine needle. Allow sufficient time for it to act, then inject more, insinuating the needle between the vein and the overlying skin to aid the separation.

2. Make a small incision over the vein, parallel to the tension lines. Gently open the incision, taking care not to tear the vein, then separate it from the tissues until you have encircled it. Pass a fine absorbable ligature round it, using a curved haemostat or aneurysm needle and tie it off.

3. As an alternative to ligature, you may avulse the vein after freeing it. Clamp a haemostat across it, and then rotate it on its long axis so that the vein is dragged into the wound and wrapped round the forceps. Close the skin with fine absorbable stitches or adherent strips.

> ### Key point
>
> - Before operating on varicose veins, ensure that you have performed the appropriate tests, that you are thoroughly familiar with the anatomy and that the veins are carefully marked.

Saphenofemoral ligation

Saphenofemoral ligation, described in 1890 by the great German surgeon from Leipzig, Friedrich Trendelenburg, disconnects the long saphenous system from the common femoral vein. To facilitate the procedure by emptying the leg veins, he placed the patient head down, feet up – now called the 'Trendelenburg position'.

1. Through an incision placed just below the groin crease, isolate, doubly ligate and divide the tributaries entering the proximal long saphenous vein.

2. Now identify and clear the saphenofemoral junction. Doubly ligate the saphenous vein flush with the femoral vein; for extra safety use a suture ligature. Make sure that there is no constriction of the femoral vein (Fig. 5.26). Apply a ligature 1 cm distally. Divide the saphenous vein between the proximal double ligature and the single distal ligature.

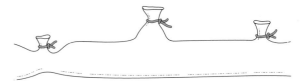

Fig. 5.26 Tying off side branches of a large vein that will remain as a conduit or be transferred to replace or bypass an arterial block. On the left the ligature is tied too close to the main channel, constricting it. In the middle the side branch is tied off too distally, leaving a cul de sac. On the right the main channel lumen remains constant.

Saphenous vein stripping in the thigh

This may be carried out after completing the saphenofemoral ligation.

1. Make a small incision in the ligated lower cut end of the proximal saphenous vein through which to pass down the end of the stripper wire or plastic leader. Apply a loose ligature to control bleeding.

2. Advance the leader until you can feel it through the skin below and medial to the knee.

3. Make a small incision 6–8 cm below the knee joint, over the vein. Apply two untied ligatures 1 cm apart.

4. Withdraw the end of the stripper above the lower ligature, which can then be tied. Loosely tie the upper ligature around the guide wire above the tip. Now

transect the vein above the first ligature, leaving the end of the guide wire projecting from the upper cut end. Gently draw on the guide wire until the stripper head is closely against the upper free end of the vein.

5. Elevate the limb and, if possible, apply compression bandages. In a controlled fashion, draw the guide wire down to strip out and concertina the vein until it emerges at the below knee incision (Fig. 5.27).

6. Squeeze out the blood by 'milking' it along the track of the stripped vein. Roll a sterile crepe bandage from the start point progressively towards the extraction wound.

7. Finally, close the incisions.

8. An alternative is to pass the stripper from below upwards – this obviates the possible difficulty of obstruction by the valves to the passage of the stripper.

ARTERIAL REPLACEMENT WITH VEIN

Vein is a frequently used replacement for diseased peripheral and coronary arteries. A segment may be carefully removed, the tributaries carefully tied off to avoid narrowing it, and it is inserted after reversing it so that the valves do not impede the flow. In the leg a segment of saphenous vein can be used in situ, after passing a special instrument to destroy the valves, and united to the artery above and below the blockage to bypass it.

ARTERIES – DIRECT PROCEDURES

During arterial procedures it may be necessary to inject or apply local topical heparin; in this case make up 500 ml isotonic saline containing 5000 IU to instil locally.

INCISION AND CLOSURE

1. First isolate the artery and obtain control using encircling tapes, untied ligatures, Silastic® tubing or placed but not tightened clamps.

2. Longitudinal incision and closure is usually suitable for medium-sized arteries but would seriously narrow smaller vessels, since eversion of the edges to obtain intimal contact increases the narrowing. Large vessels can be incised longitudinally and transversely without seriously narrowing them.

DIRECT CATHETERIZATION

This can carried out on the exposed, intact artery, which can be cannulated or catheterized directly, either proximally or distally. First ensure that you have proximal and distal control. A wide-bore artery may be opened transversely but use a longitudinal incision for a narrow vessel. Insert the tip of the catheter and relax the controlling tape, tube or clamp while fully advancing the catheter.

Fig. 5.27 Principles of vein stripping. **A** After transecting the vein on the left, pass the leader through the vein. On the right the vein has again been transected so that the leader can emerge and be brought out of the wound. **B** After ensuring that the stripper head lies safely in the subcutaneous tissues, exert traction on the leader in a controlled manner, drawing it to the right. **C** The segment of vein emerges, concertina'd on the stripper, on the right.

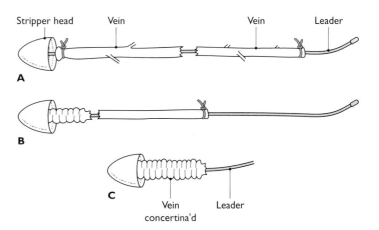

EMBOLECTOMY

A typical need for direct cannulation is for the insertion of a balloon catheter, invented by the American surgeon Fogarty (while he was still a medical student), to remove an embolus or clot, for example in a peripheral artery.

1. Fully heparinize the patient.

2. Control the vessel proximally and distally. Pass the catheter first proximally and then distally and withdraw it after gently inflating the balloon to fill the lumen and act as an extractor. As the catheterization is extended distally, use finer catheters.

3. Inject heparin in saline into the cleared vessels, before closing them and releasing the clamps or tapes.

VEIN PATCH

- This offers a valuable means of avoiding serious narrowing of the lumen when closing a longitudinal incision in an artery.
- The patch must smoothly and slightly enlarge the diameter of the vessel. If it is too small it will not have achieved the object of inserting it. If it is too big it will so enlarge the lumen as to cause turbulence and possibly result in clotting and intimal hyperplasia.

1. Excise a suitable segment of peripheral vein just longer than the defect and split it longitudinally to form a flat sheet. Trim one end to form a rounded ellipse that will fit into one end of the incision. Take a double-needled suture of suitable size and insert both needles side by side through the elliptical cut end of the graft from outside into the lumen (Fig. 5.28). Bring them from inside to the outside, just beyond and on each side of one end of the incision, so that the suture is halved. When the suture is tied it initiates an everting effect.

2. Continue from here, taking one needled thread along the back wall, one on the front wall as continuous over-and-over sutures. Each stitch passes in through the patch, out through the arterial wall. On the back wall you may need to suture from near to far; as a beginner be willing to change sides in order to sew from far to near. The flexibility of the vein patch makes it relatively easy to ensure that there is sufficient eversion to achieve intimal contact. As you reach the half-way point, leave the sutures on either side, while ensuring that the tension on them is not slackened, and direct your attention to the open end.

3. Trim the end of the vein patch into a rounded ellipse to fit into the remaining defect. Carry on inserting sutures on the back wall until you have rounded the end and continue on to meet the

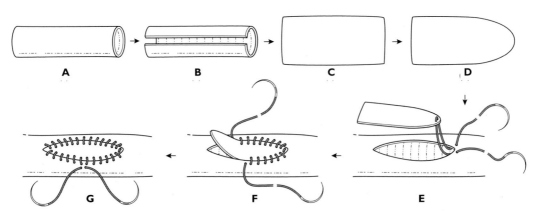

Fig. 5.28 Inserting a vein patch. **A** Excise a segment of peripheral vein. **B** Split it longitudinally. **C** Open it out. **D** Trim one end into a rounded ellipse. **E** Insert stitches in the patch and into the end of the arterial incision. **F** Continue round, keeping ahead on the back wall. Trim the end to fit into the remaining defect. **G** Carry the back wall suture around the end and continue to join the anterior suture, and tie them off.

anterior wall sutures. As the stitching is completed, both sutures emerge on the arterial surface and if adjacent sutures are tied together, they form an everting mattress suture. Do not insert sutures in such a manner that at the end you cannot be sure that the stitches have picked up the endothelium. If necessary, have the tension maintained up to a point about 1 cm before you reach the stitch from the other end. Insert the last three or four stitches slackly, under direct view. Now you can tighten them seriatim to the correct tension, and confidently tie the thread to that inserted from the other end.

4. An alternative method is to start on the anterior wall near one end, with a simple running stitch, and proceed around the corner on to the back wall. Continue along the back wall, trim the patch and carry the suture around the second corner, back on to the anterior wall. Insert stitches along this wall until you reach the starting stitch and tie off.

Key point

- Avoid finishing and tying the sutures at the end of an ellipse.

ANASTOMOSIS

End-to-end anastomosis

- A circular suture line results in some narrowing. This can be overcome by cutting the ends obliquely (see later, Fig. 5.33, p. 97).
- Any clot that forms on a transverse suture line impinges on the lumen through its whole circumference (see above, Fig. 5.21, p. 90).

1. When joining two arteries of equal diameter end-to-end, you can usually rotate the vessels, so enabling you to suture the circumference totally from the outside by taking one third at a time. Insert stay stitches between the two ends at intervals of one-third of the circumference (Fig. 5.29).

2. Begin by rotating the vessels in order to insert the first of a series of interrupted or continuous sutures, starting at the most inaccessible posterior

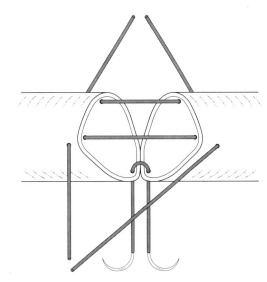

Fig. 5.29 Triangulation method of vascular anastomosis.

part. Work on both sides to come round towards the anterior surface, using the traction stitches to rotate the vessels.

3. For larger vessels it is permissible to use continuous stitches. Use unlocked stitches – they form a spiral around the circumference; because the suture is smooth and unlocked, it can accommodate to arterial pulsatile distension. As the artery distends the suture tightens, reducing the tendency for leakage at the anastomosis.

4. For small vessels and in children, use interrupted stitches. In small vessels the everting effect of continuous stitches narrows the anastomosis. In children the continuous spiral restricts arterial growth in diameter.

5. Place and tie each stitch as though you will not be able to approach it subsequently. Take care to achieve intimal contact for every stitch. Insert the stitches from outside to inside on the upstream side, from inside out on the downstream side (Fig. 5.30). If the intima is separated on the upstream side it will separate only to the anastomosis, If it is lifted on the downstream edge the dissection may spread distally.

6. The interval between stitches depends on the size of the vessels but for medium-sized arteries place them 2–3 mm apart and 2–3 mm from the edges.

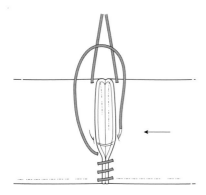

Fig. 5.30 When suturing an end-to-end anastomosis with a continuous running or interrupted stitch, insert the needle from without in on the upstream side, from within out on the downstream side. The arrow shows the direction of flow.

7. Aim to finish on the superficial face and insert the last few stitches before tying them, while ensuring that the intima is caught on each side. Only then carefully tighten them seriatim. When you are sure that every suture is perfectly placed, carefully tie them.

8. If it is not possible to mobilize and rotate the arterial ends, first insert the posterior stitches under direct vision (Fig. 5.31).

9. If necessary, leave the vessels apart, use a continuous, unlocked, double-needled suture then tighten the stitches seriatim, starting with the posterior central stitch and working outwards al-

ternately on each side towards the most recently inserted ones, then continue round to the front. Ensure that every one has a perfect grasp of the intima. This is the 'parachute' technique (Fig. 5.32). You can then continue on to the sides until the suture lines meet at the front.

10. In some situations it is valuable to cut each end obliquely (Fig. 5.33), carrying the suture line partially along the vessels, so that the incursion of the suture line into the lumen is less localized.

End-to-side anastomosis

When joining arteries, take care to avoid narrowing the lumen and also aim to reduce turbulence to a minimum. One method to achieve this is to make the anastomosis oblique, not at right angles, and also to make the anastomosis about twice the length of the arterial diameter.

1. Cut a longitudinal opening in the recipient artery approximately twice the length of its diameter. Slit the end of the tributary artery to open it, and shape it to fit the opening in the main artery (Fig. 5.34).

2. Insert one needle of a double-needled suture from inside out on the tributary 'heel', the other needle from inside out on the heel of the recipient. Proceed from here on both sides towards the toe. Prefer to insert stitches on the posterior wall first so that you can view the internal suture and ensure that it picks up the intima every time, before commencing the anterior stitching. Stop when you

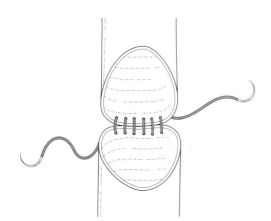

Fig. 5.31 End-to-end suture of fixed vessels starting on the back wall, identifying and picking up the full thickness including the intima in every stitch, and working towards the front.

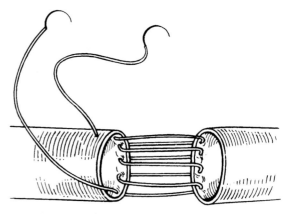

Fig. 5.32 Continuous suture anastomosis using the 'parachute' technique of placing the back wall sutures while the ends lie at a distance, then tighten the threads to bring the ends together.

Fig. 5.33 Two small vessels are united after slitting the ends and opening them out to create a wide anastomosis.

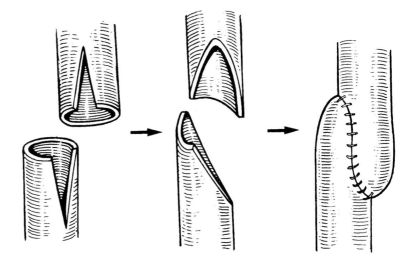

Fig. 5.34 A small vessel has been slit before joining it into the side of another vessel. The first stitch, a double-needled thread, unites the graft heel to the proximal opening in the recipient vessel. Unite the graft toe to the distal end of the opening with a second double needled thread. The back edges are first united. Stitch from each end so the back wall stitches from each end meet in the middle. Stitch the anterior wall in a similar manner.

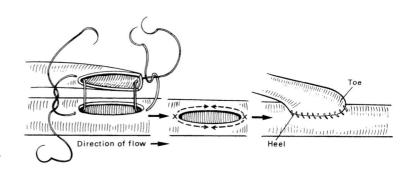

Direction of flow →

Toe

Heel

have reached the halfway point towards the toe on the posterior and anterior walls.

3. Trim the toe of the tributary vessel to fit the remaining defect.

4. Now insert one needle of a double-needled suture from inside out, just posterior to the end of the toe, and the other needle from inside to out in the corresponding end of the longitudinal hole in the recipient. Insert with great care the sutures around the extremity of the toe under vision. Suture the posterior wall up to the sutures running from the heel and tie the posterior suture, then complete the anastomosis along the front wall.

 Key point

- The critical points are at the heel and toe.

MICROVASCULAR SURGERY

- Take every opportunity to gain experience with magnification techniques. Over the years the instruments, materials and success rate for vascular surgical operations have all improved. The instruments have become finer, the suture materials and needles have become finer and smoother, and the techniques have been refined. As a result vascular surgeons can confidently operate on smaller and smaller vessels. The trend will undoubtedly continue.
- You do not need to undertake microsurgery to benefit from acquiring the techniques.
- When you have the opportunity, examine a standard vascular anastomosis using magnification.

Fig. 5.35 A loupe fitting on to a spectacle frame provides you with magnified central vision and wide normal peripheral vision.

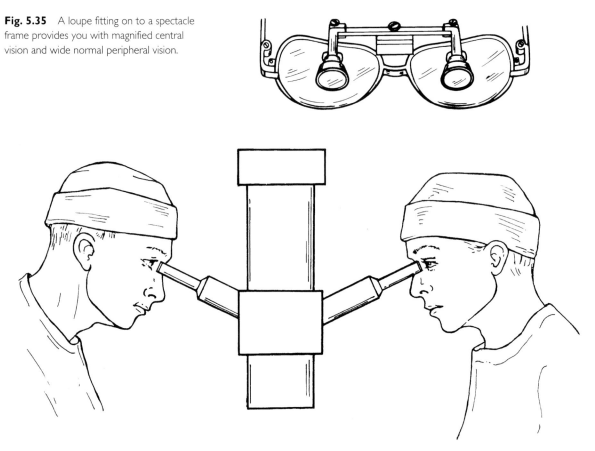

Fig. 5.36 Binocular operating microscope provides shadowless illumination. Operator and assistant can view simultaneously.

What looked very neat is likely to appear coarsely fashioned.
- The main advantage you will gain from experiencing microsurgery is that it will encourage you to aspire to gentleness and fine perfection.

1. The simplest form of magnification is a loupe (a French word with two disparate meanings – a knob, or a magnifying glass). It may be fitted to a spectacle frame (Fig. 5.35). Try the effect of performing a procedure with the naked eye and compare it with a similar one carried out while wearing the loupe. You will be impressed by the greater accuracy you achieve with magnification.

2. Higher magnification is achieved using an operating microscope (Fig. 5.36). Ordinary instruments appear crude using this, so special instruments have been devised (Fig. 5.37)

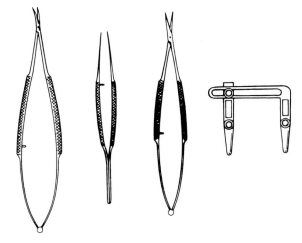

Fig. 5.37 Microsurgical scissors, dissecting forceps and needle-holder. On the right is a vascular clamp.

3. Blood vessels of 1 mm diameter or less can be anastomosed with nearly 100% success. They are conveniently held in apposition using gentle microvascular clamps (Fig. 5.38). Dissect off a cuff of adventitia, since any tags falling into the lumen attract platelets and provoke thrombosis (Fig. 5.39). Intimal damage inevitably generates

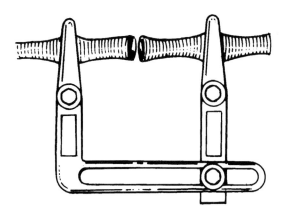

Fig. 5.38 Bring the vessel ends together, held by the double clamp.

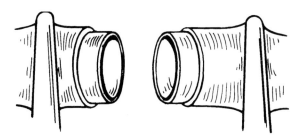

Fig. 5.39 Trim back the adventitia.

clotting. Never grasp it with forceps; instead manipulate the vessels by grasping the media. You cannot produce eversion, so join the vessels end to end. Insert a suture through the anterior wall, ensuring that it does not pick up the posterior wall. Pick up the other anterior wall and tie the suture just to appose but not constrict or distort the continuity (Fig. 5.40). Use interrupted sutures. Space stitches every 0.3 mm in arteries, 0.6 mm in veins, with three or four on each side. After completing the anterior wall, flip over the clamp to expose what had been the posterior wall and repeat the procedure. Irrigate the vessel throughout with heparin in Ringer's solution, 1000 units in 100 ml. When the anastomosis is complete you may irrigate it with 0.5% bupivacaine. Remove the distal clamp and then the proximal clamp. Gently lift the vessel, slightly obstructing it and watch for a 'flicker' as blood flows across the constriction, confirming the patency. Apply local, gentle pressure for a few minutes if there is a leak. Occasionally you will need to insert an extra stitch after reclamping the vessel and washing out any blood adhering to the edges.

 Key point

- If there is no flow, remove a couple of stitches, carefully wash out any clot and re-suture it. If there is still no flow, carefully excise the ends and start again

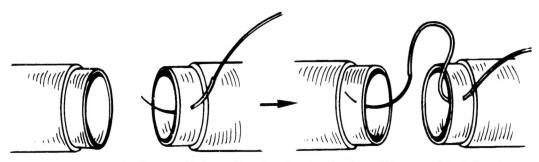

Fig. 5.40 Penetrate the vessel wall on one side from without in and on the other from within out, ready to tie the suture apposing the two edges.

4. If you wish to create an end-to-side anastomosis, excise an ellipse in the side of the recipient vessel one-third wider than the end of the vessel that will enter it.

5. Nerves can be accurately united using similar microsurgical techniques; fallopian tubes and vasa deferentes can also be reconstructed in a similar manner.

6

Handling skin
with Michael Brough

Tension lines
Inflammation
Analgesia
Wounds
Incision
Closure
Excision of skin
Excision of intradermal or subcutaneous cyst
Closing defects
Grafts
Flaps

- Skin is our interface with the outer world.
- Skin is unforgiving if it is overstretched, crushed, deprived of blood supply, irradiated.
- Elasticity gradually disappears in old age and disease.
- The skin scar is the only part of an operation seen by the patient – who judges your skill by what is visible.

TENSION LINES

Try to make and repair incisions in the line of skin tension; these run circumferentially around joint lines (Fig. 6.1). They usually run at right angles to subcutaneous muscles on the face but can best be identified by asking the patient to grimace.

INFLAMMATION

1. Inflamed skin appears red, feels hot and is swollen from the accumulation of extracellular fluid.

2. In the presence of diffuse cellulitis the surface is tethered at hair follicles and the orifices of sweat glands, producing a pitted appearance like orange peel.

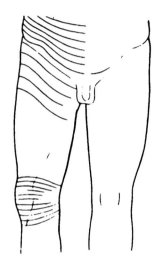

Fig. 6.1 Tension lines tend to run parallel to the creases seen at joints.

3. A localized abscess stretches the skin, producing a shiny, raised, red, hot swelling. The tension blanches the crown of the swelling, which becomes necrotic as the abscess 'points', goes black and may rupture.

ANALGESIA

1. If local anaesthesia is unlikely to suffice on its own, consider, as an alternative to general anaesthesia, giving premedication with systemic analgesics (G *an* = not + *algeein* = to feel pain) – but this is appropriate only if you have full facilities for resuscitation and postoperative recovery.

2. Always have adrenaline (epinephrine) 1:1000 and hydrocortisone 100 mg available in case the patient develops an allergic or other reaction.

3. Lidocaine (lignocaine) and prilocaine in a concentration of 4% is effective when applied

topically on mucous membranes but is ineffective on the skin. However, consider applying it topically into open wounds or instilling it into the pleural or peritoneal cavities, joint spaces and fracture sites. Lidocaine (lignocaine) 25 mg and prilocaine 25 mg in 1 g of cream (EMLA®) applied 1.5–3 g/cm² for a minimum of 2 hours under an occlusive dressing is usually effective in producing skin analgesia.

4. Local infiltration anaesthesia is a simple and safe method of producing a limited area of analgesia. Lidocaine (lignocaine) 0.5–2.0% can be injected up to a maximum of 3 mg/kg body weight and its effect lasts up to 90 minutes. A maximum of 7 mg/kg can be injected with 1:200 000 adrenaline to cause vasoconstriction, reducing bleeding and slowing absorption. Bupivacaine injected in concentrations of up to 0.5% with a maximum dose of 2 mg/kg body weight produces up to 12 hours of analgesia. It takes several minutes to take effect; lignocaine 1% and bupivacaine 0.5% may be mixed in equal volumes to overcome this. Ropivacaine 0.75% may be safer than bupivacaine.

5. First raise an intracutaneous bleb, using a fine needle away from a sensitive or inflamed area. Wait for it to take effect then inject through it intracutaneously along the line of the proposed incision, to produce a raised ridge resembling orange peel. Now infiltrate deeper, using a longer and larger needle, keeping the point moving as you inject, to minimize the danger of injecting into a vein.

6. Do not inject under high pressure, especially in the presence of inflammation. It is painful and the pressure of fluid will restrict the blood supply, as will the addition of adrenaline. A notorious risk when infiltrating a ring of local anaesthetic around the base of a finger is to raise the circumferential pressure and may result in finger necrosis. Always inject proximally at the level of the interphalangeal

---

> ### 🔑 Key point
>
> - Do not begin the procedure until the anaesthetic has had time to act. You undermine the confidence of the patient if your initial act causes pain. Wait a minimum of 2 minutes, but preferably wait for 5 minutes.

web. The risk can be further reduced by adding 1500 units of hyaluronidase, which aids the rapid spread of the anaesthetic within the tissues.

WOUNDS

- From the history of the injury, sedulous clinical examination and, if necessary, appropriate imaging, assess the damage before starting the repair. Determine whether there is damage to nerves, vessels, bones, tendons and soft tissues; in penetrating injuries, look for exit wounds. Do not, though, blindly explore the wound if you intend to open it up at operation for fear of causing further injury.
- Remember that many injuries have legal, compensation and insurance implications, so immediately make careful notes, drawings and photographs if possible.

1. Under sterile conditions carefully and, if necessary, widely clean and prepare the area.

2. Explore the wound with fingers and probes, extending it when appropriate.

3. Completely stop bleeding.

4. Assiduously clean the wound. Irrigate it with plenty of sterile saline. In the presence of contamination, use only mild, water-based antiseptics; strong ones damage the tissues. Take time to remove all the dead and foreign material. If you leave ingrained dirt, healing is prejudiced, as the resultant scar may remain pigmented.

5. Search for and remove all foreign material and dead tissue.

6. Search for and identify deeper damage to vessels, nerves, muscles, bones and joints. Do not hesitate to enlarge the incision in these circumstances. If you do need to extend the wound in a cosmetically important area, consider following the tension lines. Carry out appropriate repair of deep tissues before deciding whether or not to close the skin.

7. Finally, recheck haemostasis, repeat the irrigation of the tissues and once more check for foreign material and dead or ischaemic tissue.

8. Unless the wound is clean, tidy, looks healthy and has recently been acquired, do not close it. Leave it open and determine to carry out delayed primary closure when it is healthy.

9. If there is skin loss, loosely maintain the tissues in their correct position and defer attempts at reconstruction. If you are experienced you may cover a clean wound with a split skin graft (see p. 109).

10. If the wound is safe to close but irregular and sited in a cosmetically important place such as the face, take the greatest care to align the skin correctly to avoid producing a distorted scar.

 Key point

- Do not attempt immediate primary closure of doubtful wounds. In the presence of delayed presentation, trauma, contamination, foreign material or ischaemia and tissue loss, be prepared to monitor the wound for 24–48 hours to allow you to exclude infection or impending necrosis, and allow oedema to settle, then carry out delayed primary closure. Do not attempt to close the wound under tension.

INCISION

1. Decide the line and depth of the incision, taking into account the primary purpose of the procedure but secondarily considering the cosmetic effects, including the direction of the tension lines. If the incision will be complicated, first mark matching points with 'Bonney's blue' dye (Victor Bonney, London gynaecologist 1872–1953) so that you can accurately appose them during closure.

2. Stretch and fix the skin at the starting point using the non-dominant hand (Fig. 6.2).

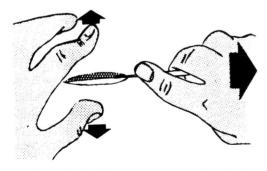

Fig. 6.2 Steady the skin using the fingers and thumb of your non-dominant hand.

3. Except when a short stab wound is required, use the belly of the knife and draw it along the line of the incision, rather than pressing it in statically. Cut to an even depth throughout so that you can use the whole length of the wound. Do not leave half-incised ends.

4. When possible, cut boldly with a single sweep of the knife. Tentative scratches detach pieces that will undergo necrosis and delay healing (Fig. 6.3). Occasionally, scissors are preferable to a scalpel for cutting loose flaps, provided the blades are rigid and remain in contact; if they separate, the skin will be crushed and 'chewed'. Cut perpendicular to the surface to avoid slicing it.

5. Control initial oozing from the cut edges by pressing with your finger tips along one edge while your assistant presses on the opposite side (Fig. 6.4).

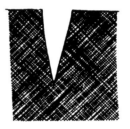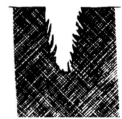

Fig. 6.3 Make smooth incisions. The diagram demonstrates this on the left; on the right, multiple cuts produce ragged incisions with tags that will die and delay healing.

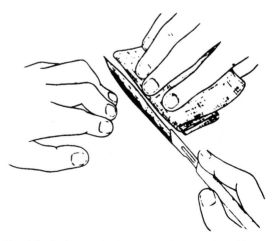

Fig. 6.4 Reduce oozing by compressing one edge with your non-dominant fingers while your assistant compresses the other side. You may spread the pressure with a flattened swab.

Use folded gauze swabs if necessary. Diminish severe oozing by applying haemostatic forceps at intervals of about 1 cm to the dermal edges – not the epidermis – and lay the forceps handles on to the intact surface to evert the edges (Fig. 6.5). Never place haemostatic forceps on the epidermis. This crushes the skin and produces ugly scarring. You may identify and pick up individual vessels with fine artery forceps, twist them and release them. Avoid ligatures close to the skin surface. Use diathermy current sparingly since skin burns heal slowly; pick up the vessel with fine forceps, apply 'cutting' current at the lowest intensity for the minimal time. Bipolar diathermy is safer than monopolar diathermy, since the current passes only between the two forceps tips and does not heat surrounding tissues.

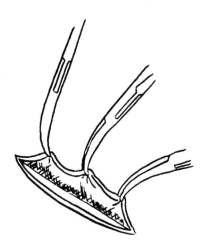

Fig. 6.5 Control bleeding from the wound edge, especially on the scalp, by attaching haemostatic forceps to the dermis and using them to evert the skin.

CLOSURE

Simple linear

1. Close a simple incision by accurately re-apposing the living skin edges. To avoid any displacement of the edges of a straight incision, insert skin hooks at each end and have them gently distracted by an assistant while you insert the stitches.

2. Healing cannot take place if the dead, keratinized surface cells are apposed by inverting the edges. It is preferable to err on the side of slight eversion (Fig. 6.6).

3. Place the stitches within a few millimetres of the edges.

4. In the past, hand-held straight needles were popular for skin closure but the risk of needle-stick injury has forced us to convert to indirectly controlled curved needles held in needle-holders. Use cutting needles mounted with fine thread. Silk has for many years been the standard material but in recent years fine monofilament polyamide or polypropylene have become popular and are claimed to cause minimal tissue reaction, especially for closing wounds on the face.

5. Grip the needle in the needle-holder on the swaged side of the middle. Fully pronate your hand so that the needle point enters perpendicular to the skin surface from the dominant side to emerge on the non-dominant side, or from the far side to near. As you progressively supinate your hand, drive the needle along the path of its curve, emerging in the wound. Capture it and reinsert it into the other side exactly opposite the point of emergence and at exactly the same depth. As the point emerges at the skin level, once more capture it, further supinating your hand to draw it through (Fig. 6.7). To aid the passage of the needle, gently apply counterpressure with closed dissecting forceps or use skin hooks to evert the skin edges.

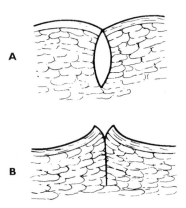

Fig. 6.6 **A** The skin edges are inverted, achieving contact only between the dead keratinized surfaces. **B** The edges are slightly everted; the living edges are in contact and can unite.

Fig. 6.7 Use a skin hook (left) or closed dissecting forceps (right) to evert the skin edges. Press closed forceps a short distance from the edge, or use them to push back the edge to produce eversion. Make sure that the needle crosses between the edges at exactly the same depth. If you grab the skin with forceps you will crush it and cause scarring.

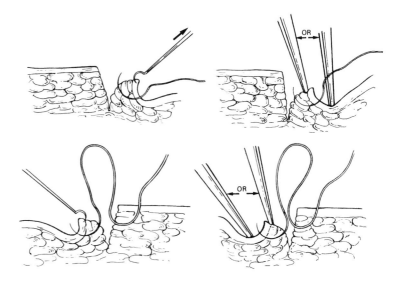

6. If the skin has a tendency to invert, use an everting mattress stitch (Fig. 6.8).

7. As important as the insertion of the suture is the tying and placing of the knot. Tie the knot just tightly enough to appose the edges. If you tie it too tightly it will produce a ladder scar. Site the knot to one side of the closure.

8. Remove sutures on the face after 3–4 days, after 7–10 days in abdominal and similar wound closures.

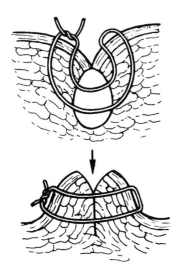

Fig. 6.8 Everting mattress suture will correct the tendency for the skin to invert.

Subcuticular stitch

1. An excellent alternative to conventional stitching is the subcuticular stitch, avoiding stitch marks on the skin. Use it only if there is no tension, or if you have overcome the tension by inserting deeper stitches first. Suitable smooth, non-absorbable material is monofilamentous polyamide, polypropylene or polyethylene.

2. Introduce the suture in the line of the wound about 1 cm from one end, into the extreme end of the wound. Insert stitches on alternate sides into the intradermal layer all at the same depth, each one crossing the gap at right angles to avoid distorting the skin (Fig. 6.9).

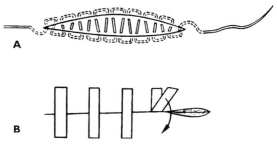

A

B

Fig. 6.9 Skin closure. **A** Subcuticular stitch: when the stitch ends are distracted, the edges are drawn together. The stitch may be absorbable and can be left, or non-absorbable and can be withdrawn. **B** Provided the wound is absolutely dry you may appose the edges using adherent strips of tape.

3. At the far end, drive the stitch to emerge on the skin about 1 cm beyond the end in the line of the incision.

4. The intradermal stitches lie parallel to the skin surfaces. It is necessary to have the needle-holder exactly perpendicular to the undisturbed skin surface, in order to drive the curved needle in its jaws along a path parallel to the skin surface. Moreover, since you will stitch alternately to one side, then the other, you will need to change the needle to point towards and away from you with each stitch. However, if you evert the skin using a skin hook or apply pressure with closed dissecting forceps, you can distort the skin edges, allowing you to insert the needle with ease (Fig. 6.10). Do not use your fingers for fear of sustaining a needle prick.

5. Having inserted all the stitches, now distract the suture ends to straighten it, thus drawing the skin edges together. Maintain tension on the ends either by clamping on lead or other metal clips to the emerging threads or by taping them down to the skin. When the wound is healed, release the tethering, pull each end in turn to free the thread, then cut one end and pull the remainder of the intact thread out from the other end. If the wound is long there is a danger that the suture will break when you try to pull it through in one piece; to avoid this, break it up into lengths of about 5–6 cm by bringing it to the surface and knotting it (Fig. 6.11).

6. You can insert absorbable material so that it does not need to be removed. Insert a subcuticular stitch at one end of the incision, picking up both sides, and tie it. Proceed from here along the wound inserting subcuticular stitches on alternate sides until you reach the far end. You may now tie a knot after taking a stitch through both sides. This may be difficult to do. Alternatively, bring out the needle about 1 cm from the end of the wound to one side, return the needle back through the same hole to emerge within the wound. Reinsert it into the wound to emerge about 1 cm from the end on the other side and back again. Finally bring it to the surface and cut it off flush with the skin (Fig. 6.11). This offers sufficient fixation.

One of us (MB) starts by inserting and gently tying a simple, looped, linear stitch in the line of, but clear of, one end of the incision. Reinsert the stitch between the looped and tied stitch and the end of the incision. Now stitch back and forth to complete the subcuticular suture. At the far end, insert the stitch to emerge in the line of, but clear of the end of, the wound. Adjust the tension to appose the wound edges. Take a final stitch away from, but in the line of, the incision and gently tie the end to the exposed emerged segment of suture. Thus the

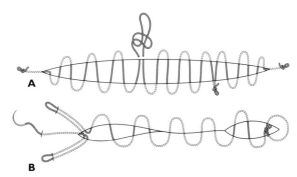

Fig. 6.11 Two tips when inserting subcuticular stitches. **A** When inserting a long non-absorbable stitch, H.S. Tantawy of Cairo suggests coming to the surface every 5–6 cm, tying a slip knot, reinserting the needle into the same hole and tightening the knot down to the skin. A similar technique suffices to fix the ends. Withdraw the stitch in segments between the slip knots. **B** There are several choices for securing the ends of an absorbable subcuticular stitch. On the right, insert an encircling subcuticular stitch and tie it within the wound. On the left, bring the needle out to the surface at an angle, return it through the same hole, repeat this at another angle and finally bring it out and cut it flush.

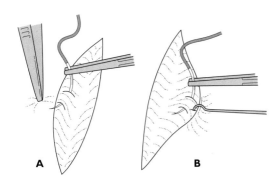

Fig. 6.10 Subcuticular stitch. By everting the skin edges you can insert stitches that will be parallel to the skin surface when the eversion is relaxed. Produce eversion either by pressing with the closed tips of dissecting forceps as shown in **A**, or traction from a skin hook as shown in **B**.

incision and the stitching at both ends form a straight line. The sutured wound can be exposed and washed. To remove the stitch, simply cut the looped thread at each end and withdraw the buried stitch from one end.

7. Adhesive strips also offer an alternative to conventional stitches to appose skin edges (Fig. 6.9). Unless they adhere right up to the skin edges, they have an inverting effect, so ensure that there is no oozing, that the skin is completely dry. If possible, first apply an adhesive such as tincture of benzoin and allow it to dry.

8. Skin staples are sometimes used as an alternative to stitches (see Ch. 2, p. 14). As a trainee, take every opportunity to practise stitching. It is the most versatile method of joining soft tissues. Reserve staples for exceptional circumstances when these will be of benefit to the patient.

EXCISION OF SKIN

1. When excising skin that is diseased, scarred, traumatized, ischaemic or adherent to a lesion that must be completely excised, plan it carefully, if necessary marking the incision with Bonney's blue. Take into account the site – facial skin has an excellent blood supply and heals well, palmar skin of the hands and plantar skin of the feet is specialized and cannot be replaced with skin of equal quality and nerve supply. Elderly patients often have mobile spare skin.

2. When excising circular lesions, plan an elliptical incision, lying along the tension lines, with pointed ends (Fig. 6.12). The wider the ellipse, the longer it should be, or the resulting scar will be ugly.

3. Many of these lesions are amenable to excision under local anaesthesia. In the absence of infection, tend to use a dilute solution, with added adrenaline (epinephrine), that can be infiltrated widely over the extent of the lesion to reduce oozing.

4. Excise benign lesions with minimal margins but remove malignant and potentially recurrent lesions with adequate margins both laterally and in depth.

5. Make the incision while keeping the scalpel blade perpendicular to the skin surface to avoid

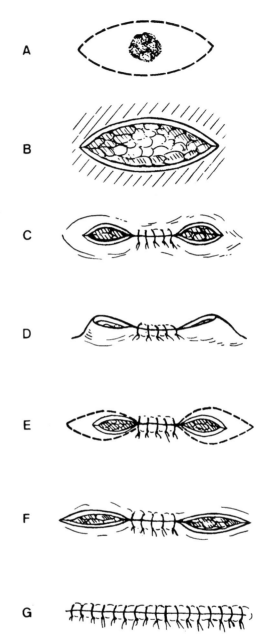

Fig. 6.12 **A** Excise a circular lesion using an elliptical incision with pointed ends, if necessary first marking the incision with ink. **B** Be prepared to undermine the skin edges if this will help closure. **C** Close the central part first. **D** This often produces raised 'dog ears' at each end. **E** Carefully outline the bases of the dog ears and excise them as in **F**. **G** Finally close the slightly longer but flat wound.

slicing it. In some areas, such as the skin near the eyelids of young people, this may cause distortion and a local flap may provide a better cosmetic result.

6. Close an elliptical incision (Fig. 6.12) after undermining the skin on either side. In order to appose the edges accurately it may be convenient to start in the middle, working outwards. 'Dog ears' may mar the appearance of the scar, although undermining the skin beyond the ends of the incision, as well as at the sides, reduces them. If they are unsightly, mark out the base and excise them to achieve a straight, flat scar.

EXCISION OF INTRADERMAL OR SUBCUTANEOUS CYST

1. This can be excised under local anaesthesia. You rarely need to shave the hair.

2. Carefully raise an intracutaneous bleb at the edge of the swelling. Through this inject dilute, say 0.5% lidocaine (lignocaine) intracutaneously over the top and around but not into the cyst. The volume of anaesthetic separates the cyst from the surrounding tissues.

3. Do not rush to make the incision. Allow about 5 minutes for the local anaesthetic to take effect.

4. Place the incision just off centre of the punctum or summit of the swelling, otherwise you risk entering the cyst.

5. Achieve haemostasis by identifying the small intradermal vessels and catching them with fine haemostats. The vessels lie in the subcuticular layer, not in the epithelium, so avoid catching this. As a rule, it is sufficient to leave on the haemostats until you are ready to close but one or two may need to be ligated with the finest absorbable material. If you intend to use diathermy coagulation, set it at the lowest effective setting and use it for the minimum time. If you burn the epithelium it will produce a visible scar.

6. Identify the cyst wall, work around it and gradually free it without rupturing it. Avoid grasping it with forceps. The last portion to free should be the punctum, attached to the skin surface; if necessary excise a small ellipse to avoid puncturing it.

7. If you rupture the cyst, carefully identify all the lining and excise it to prevent a recurrence.

8. After securing haemostasis, suture the skin.

9. As an alternative to a dressing, apply a varnish skin spray.

CLOSING DEFECTS

1. Do not pull together skin edges under tension and expect them to heal.

2. In some cases the skin edges will not come together, not because there is a skin deficiency but because of deficiency of the attached deep layers. You may transfer tension from the skin to the deeper layers by drawing them together first and then closing the skin without tension.

3. Undercutting the skin is of value only if it is the deep attachments that prevent the edges from being drawn together (Fig. 6.13). If the skin is already tight do not expect to succeed – the freed skin edges may merely retract further. Relatively avascular skin must retain its blood supply by including the subdermal plexus within the subcutaneous fat. Evert the skin first with dissecting forceps and later with the fingers (Fig. 6.14).

4. When the lengths of the edges of a defect are incongruous, insert guide stitches that will later be removed. Place the first of these into the middle of each of the edges, and place others halving the intervening space (Fig. 6.15), and so on. Now insert the definitive stitches and then remove the guide stitches. In this way you can spread the difference in length of the edges evenly.

5. If it is important to close a defect to provide skin cover, for example over a bony fracture, it may be

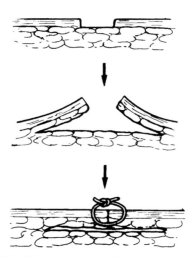

Fig. 6.13 If the skin is tethered but elastic, free it so that the edges can be apposed.

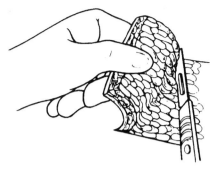

Fig. 6.14 While undercutting the skin, evert it so you keep in the right plane.

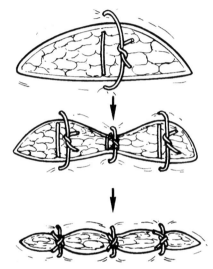

Fig. 6.15 If the length of the edges of the defect are incongruous insert a stitch that joins the middle of each edge, then halve the space on each side and so on. When you have inserted the definitive stitches, remove the guide stitches. In this way you spread the difference in length evenly.

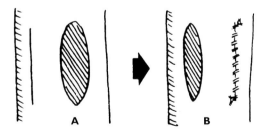

Fig. 6.16 **A** A defect that must be covered with good-quality skin; to the left of the defect a relaxing incision has been made. **B** The bridge of skin between the relaxing incision and the defect has been mobilized and slid across to cover the defect. The resulting gap could be closed with a split -kin graft.

necessary to create a relaxing incision so that the adjacent skin can be slid across to close the defect (Fig. 6.16). Do not embark on such a procedure unless you have special training. Inexpert management will prejudice survival of the skin cover.

6. The most generally effective temporary measure is to apply a split-skin graft.

GRAFTS

1. The name is said to arise from the fact that shoots cut for grafting trees resembled a stylus or pen with which to write (= G *graphein*). Its surgical use implies tissue that is totally freed and placed elsewhere, deriving its nourishment from the tissue bed in which it is placed.

2. Grafts can be harvested under general or local anaesthesia. If you use local anaesthesia, consider first applying a cream containing lidocaine (lignocaine) 25 mg and prilocaine 25 mg/g. Apply 1.5–3 g/cm^2 for a minimum of 2 hours beneath an occlusive dressing, over the donor area. Alternatively infiltrate the whole area with dilute – e.g. 0.25% – lidocaine (lignocaine) with 1500 units of hyalase.

3. Survival depends upon there being suitable conditions at the receptor site. These are:

a. Adequate and stable contact between donor graft and recipient site. This implies that there is no separation because of graft movement, interposed necrotic or foreign material, slough, exudation, haematoma or seroma,

b. Adequate blood supply to establish a source of nourishment. This implies no serious ischaemic or postradiation effects at the recipient site.

c. Absence of certain types of microorganism, in particular β-haemolytic streptococcus type A, which produces fibrinolysin, thus prejudicing adherence of the graft.

Split-skin graft

1. This general purpose graft, described by Karl Thiersch of Erlangen and Leipzig in 1874, includes some germinal layers but leaves behind the hair follicles, sebaceous glands and sweat glands, which provide fresh epithelial cells to resurface the donor area, usually within 1–2 weeks.

2. Split-skin grafts may be thin, requiring minimal nourishment and therefore surviving when the blood supply is relatively poor, but are fragile and not capable of withstanding heavy wear and tear. The donor site heals rapidly, allowing the taking of further grafts – useful if extensive skin replacement is required. Thick skin grafts demand a suitable base but once established are relatively robust. The donor site heals slowly.

3. The recipient site may be fresh, as following excision of tissues including skin, or following preparation after skin loss resulting from burns, ulcers, pressure sores and other causes of skin loss.

4. Following surgical excision or traumatic skin loss, immediate skin grafting can be carried out provided the base has an adequate blood supply; fat is poorly supplied with blood vessels and makes a poor recipient base, as does bone stripped of its periosteum. Before applying a skin graft achieve absolute haemostasis, since bleeding beneath the graft prevents it from gaining nutriments and from adhering to the bed.

5. Healthy granulation tissue consisting of capillary loops and fibroblasts makes a suitable recipient base. It should be pink, fairly compact and not oedematous, with minimum exudation and no slough. Infection with most organisms except *Streptococcus pyogenes* does not usually preclude successful grafting, but take swabs for culture. If slough is present, be willing to excise it surgically. If granulation tissue does not form on a raw area this suggests that a graft is unlikely to survive.

6. Cut the graft using a Watson knife, which has an adjustable roller to control the thickness of the cut. Carefully watch an expert cut a graft and make sure you are supervised by an expert until you become competent at this procedure. Depending on the recipient site and the required extent of the graft, you may select the donor site. A common donor area is the front of the thigh. You need a flat skin surface and this is created by preceding the knife blade with a lubricated flat board held in your non-dominant hand while your assistant holds a dry board steadily applying counter pressure above the donor site to slightly stretch it and flatten it (Fig. 6.17), while supporting the

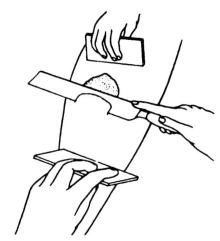

Fig. 6.17 Cutting a split-skin graft. Hold a lubricated flat board in your left hand and slowly draw it ahead of the knife held in the right hand, to flatten and stretch the skin as you cut the graft with a back and forth movement. Your assistant holds a dry, fixed board above the start of the cut to flatten, stretch and fix the skin. The assistant's other hand may lift up the soft tissues from below to expose a larger area on the upper surface.

undersurface of the limb to create the largest and flattest area possible.

7. After adjusting the roller and lubricating the undersurface of the blade, hold the graft knife flat against the skin, concentrating on smoothly drawing it back and forth in a sawing motion.

 Key point

- Do not press hard, try to advance too quickly, or angle the knife, since this will make it cut out. Try not to stop until you have completed the whole graft.

8. The graft accumulates on the knife like thin paper in folds. The donor site appears initially white, soon erupting with fine petechial haemorrhages if the graft is thin and larger drops and more prolific bleeding following a deeper cut. Too thick a graft reveals subcutaneous fat. When you have completed the cut, raise the knife to lift the curtain-like graft and cut across with scissors.

9. Lay a large graft on tulle gras, outer side (dull,

keratinized) down, living surface (shiny, deep) uppermost. Gently open out and spread the graft.

10. Pick up the tulle gras with attached graft and lay it, graft side down, onto the recipient site, allowing it to overlap the edges of the defect.

11. A popular method of fixing the graft is to insert stitches around the periphery to fix it and use these to fix a compressing dressing over it. Insert the stitches through the graft then through the skin; if you insert it first through the skin you lift off the graft (Fig. 6.18). Leave the suture long after tying it. If you cause bleeding under the graft, carefully squeeze it out and maintain compression until it stops. When the graft has been encircled with sutures place a carefully shaped cotton-wool pad over the graft and tie the ends of the stitches over it to hold it in place. Plastic surgeons often use cotton wool impregnated with flavine emulsion, or alternatively use shaped polyurethane sponge. Depending on the site and your ability to attain fixation and create even compression, you may insert stitches only or provide compression only.

12. The donor site was formerly covered with tulle gras but alginate dressing (Kaltstat®) has replaced it, since it is more comfortable. The donor site is more painful than the recipient site.

13. Power-driven dermatomes are valuable tools in expert hands when large areas of skin need to be cut.

14. Meshed grafts have several advantages. The skin is normally fed between rollers, which cut it in a pattern that allows the sheet to be extended in a net-like pattern (Fig. 6.19). If a machine is not available it is possible to create small mesh grafts using a scalpel. Meshing increases the area of the graft, valuable if there is a large defect. Its other main advantage is that any exudates, blood or pus can pass through the holes in the mesh instead of gathering under the graft and lifting it off.

15. Any spare skin graft can be stored in the refrigerator at approximately 4°C for up to 3 weeks after being wrapped in sterile, saline-moistened gauze.

Full-thickness graft

1. This was described in 1873 by John Wolfe, an Austrian ophthalmologist who settled in Glasgow. It includes all layers of the skin freed of subcutaneous tissue. Because the whole thickness of skin is used, the donor site will not heal spontaneously.

2. It is often used on the face, because the cosmetic appearance is very good if the donor site is carefully selected for thickness and colour. Favourite donor sites for replacement facial skin include postauricular, supraclavicular, antecubital and groin.

3. Because of its thickness the recipient site must be clean with a satisfactory vascular base and edges.

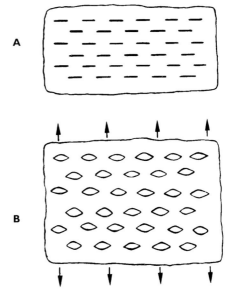

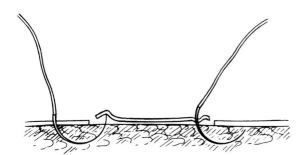

Fig. 6.18 On the left, the needle has passed first through the skin and as it pushes up through the graft it tends to lift and displace it. On the right, the needle first passes through the graft without displacing it.

Fig. 6.19 The effect of meshing the graft. **A** Make a series of cuts in the split skin graft. **B** The graft can be stretched to increase its area.

4. Make a pattern of the defect and draw it on the donor site with Bonney's blue.

5. Cut the graft with perpendicular edges, avoiding slicing them. Turn the graft and carefully cut off all the fat, since this will form a partition separating the graft from the base, depriving it of nutrition.

6. Carefully sew in the graft. As it is excised it shrinks and must be slightly stretched to normal tension to fit accurately into the new site.

7. The donor site can usually be closed as a linear scar.

FLAPS

- A flap, unlike a graft, retains its blood supply through a pedicle instead of picking up a fresh supply at the recipient area like a free graft.
- The blood supply to some flaps is haphazard and they are called 'random pattern flaps'. Because of this, the length of the base attachment is critical in relation to the length of the flap.
- It is recognized that some flaps can be much longer in relation to the base and still survive. The reason is that the blood vessels remain intact entering the base of the flap. These are called 'axial pattern flaps'.

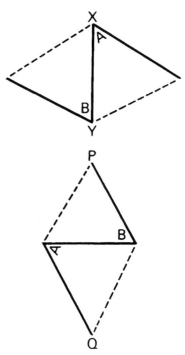

Fig. 6.20 Z-plasty. To extend the length of the line XY in the upper diagram, raise the triangular flaps marked A and B as far as the dotted lines. Transpose them and suture them in place as in the lower drawing so that the length PQ is longer than XY, at the cost of width.

Z-plasty

1. This overcomes the problem of linear shortening by taking advantage of the fact that skin is flexible and elastic; it may be shifted in from the side to increase the length of the contracture.

2. In Figure 6.20 the diamond shape at the top is wider than its height. The line XY in the top diagram represents a linear contraction. Make an incision along it. At X make an incision of the same length downwards and to the right at an angle of 60°; at Y make an incision of the same length upwards and to the left at an angle of 60°.

3. Raise the flaps with tips marked A and B on to the bases marked with broken lines.

4. Now transpose A anticlockwise on its base, rotating B anticlockwise on its base so that they cross as in the lower diagram. The diamond so formed is now taller than it is wide. The length PQ is greater than the height of the upper diamond, XY.

5. Increasing the angle of the side incisions increases the lengthening effect of the Z-plasty while decreasing the angle of the side incisions decreases the lengthening effect.

6. A series of Z-plasties may be used to increase the length of a long contracture by incorporating width along its whole length.

Transposition flaps

1. When skin is lost or excised it may not be possible to draw the edges together, or to do so may cause distortion. A variety of flaps may be used.

2. A simple transposition flap can be used to close a defect (Fig. 6.21). If a defect has to be closed, a suitably shaped flap can be raised and sewn in to close it.

3. Close the defect left by the flap as a linear suture line.

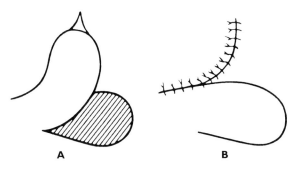

Fig. 6.21 Transposition flap. In **A** the excised area is shaded and the flap is raised. In **B** the flap has been transposed into the defect and the gap left has been closed as a linear suture line.

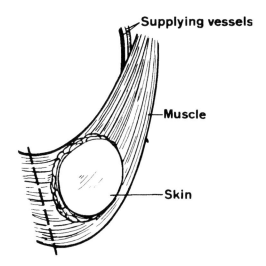

Fig. 6.22 Myocutaneous flap. The muscle has been transected along the broken line. The overlying area of skin, which derives its blood supply from the muscle, can be moved together with the muscle belly, hinging on its supplying blood vessels.

Myocutaneous flaps

1. As the understanding of the blood supply increased, advantage has been taken to improve the survival of transposed skin by bringing its blood supply with it.

2. An area of skin nourished from the underlying muscle can be moved with the body of the muscle. Some muscles – such as the latissimus dorsi – have the neurovascular bundle enter them from one end. The other end, together with an area of overlying skin, can be mobilized and swung a considerable distance to fill a defect (Fig. 6.22).

Free tissue transfer

Since the blood supply can be identified and preserved in an axial skin flap, or to a myocutaneous flap, the vessels can be divided and the whole can be transferred elsewhere. The blood vessels are joined in to local vessels, usually two veins for each artery, employing microsurgical techniques (see Ch. 5, pp. 97–100).

Tissue expansion

As an alternative to bringing in skin from elsewhere, local skin can be obtained by expanding it. This is achieved by placing a tissue expander under the fascia or muscle (Fig. 6.23). The expander is connected via a tube to a small reservoir sited subcutaneously. Over a period of time saline can be injected via the reservoir to increase its volume and expand the skin. When sufficient expansion has been achieved, the tissue expander can be removed and the spare skin is available to close a defect.

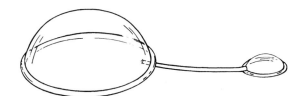

Fig. 6.23 Tissue expansion. The hemispherical expander is attached to a small reservoir. The expander is inserted subfascially or submuscularly. The subcutaneously sited reservoir can be injected transcutaneously with saline to gradually distend the expander and the overlying tissues.

7

Handling connective and soft tissues

Percutaneous diagnostic procedures
Aspiration of fluid
Cytology
Needle biopsy
Open biopsy
Connective tissue
Areolar tissue
Aponeuroses
Tendons
Ligaments
Nerves
Skeletal muscle
Cartilage
Mucoperiosteum
Soft tissues
Breast
Lymph nodes
Abdominal wall
Organs
Bowel
Liver
Spleen
Pancreas
Kidney
Ureter
Bladder
Uterus
Lung
Heart
Endocrine and other glands
Brain and spinal cord

- Each body tissue has a characteristic appearance and feel at different ages, in health and disease.
- Make sure you are familiar with the anatomy and consistency of the tissues before embarking on an operation.
- In particular, familiarize yourself with the tissue planes between the target structure and the surrounding tissues, otherwise you risk inadvertently causing damage.

PERCUTANEOUS DIAGNOSTIC PROCEDURES

Many procedures can be carried out under local anaesthesia (see Ch. 6, pp. 102–103).

ASPIRATION OF FLUID

1. Carry out the procedure under sterile conditions. Use a needle that is long enough so you do not need to insert it to the Luer connection (Luer was a German instrument-maker working in Paris); if it breaks off at the junction with the shaft, you may not be able to recapture the needle.

2. Attach a syringe and aspirate. If you obtain no fluid, try rotating the needle. Do not alter the direction of the needle except by first withdrawing it.

CYTOLOGY

1. Fine-needle aspiration cytology (FNAC) can often be carried out under local anaesthetic, although this may be unnecessary. Fix the target between the fingers of one hand while holding the syringe and needle (usually a 21 gauge) in the other.

2. When the tip is correctly sited apply suction by attempting to withdraw the piston of the syringe. Move the needle in and out in jerky reciprocal movements to detach cells, which will be drawn into the needle.

3. Simultaneous fixation of a lump, control of the needle position and aspiration of a standard syringe are difficult. A number of mechanical aids are available based on the principle shown in Figure 7.1.

4. Cell harvesting is improved if the syringe and needle are first washed out with a mixture of physiological (0.9%) saline with 1000 units of heparin. After completing the procedure, withdraw the syringe and needle and eject the contents on to several prelabelled microscope slides and immediately apply fixative to them. Finally, draw up some fixative through the needle into the syringe from a specimen bottle and empty the syringe back into the bottle. The ejected cells will be recovered by centrifugation and stained, along with those on the slides, for cytological examination. In some cases the cells are immediately smeared on to a slide, using a cover slip, air-dried and then stained.

NEEDLE BIOPSY

1. In order to confirm the histological diagnosis, grade and receptor status, and to carry out a DNA analysis of a tumour, obtain a core of tissue. Take advice beforehand from the pathologist as to how the specimen should be preserved and sent for examination.

2. If the lesion is not palpable the needle may be guided with the aid of ultrasound or radiological imaging.

3. One method is with a hollow needle such as a Tru-Cut® (Travenol). From the end of a sharp hollow needle protrudes the bevelled cutting end of a stylette. The proximal part of the stylette does not fill the lumen of the needle (Fig. 7.2).

   a. After infiltrating the skin with local anaesthetic, make a small incision with a pointed scalpel, just large enough to accept the needle. Insert the closed needle through the incision and into the lump to be biopsied, while steadying a mobile lump with the fingers of the other hand.

   b. Hold the needle still and advance the stylette further into the lump. Now hold the stylette still and advance the needle, which cuts off and encloses the tissue that bulged into the thinned section of the stylette. If the tissue is very hard, advance the closed

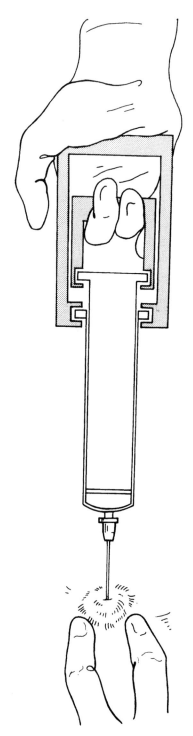

Fig. 7.1   The principle of fine-needle aspiration cytology. The action of a syringe holder allows the syringe and needle to be controlled with one hand while the other steadies the lump. Squeezing the handle of the syringe holder draws out the piston and exerts a suction effect through the attached needle.

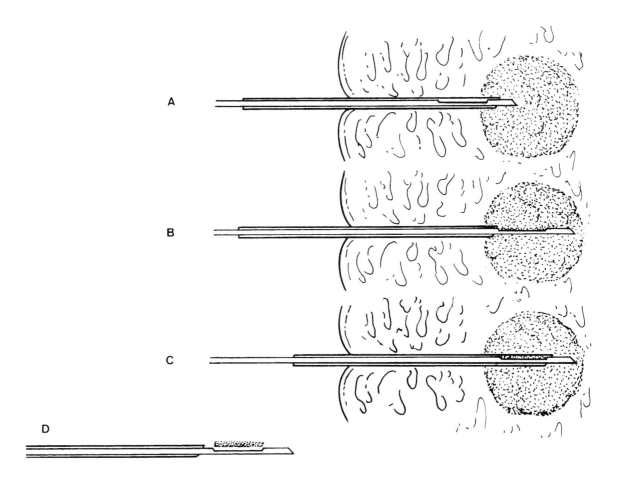

Fig. 7.2 Needle biopsy. **A** Insert the closed needle tip into the tissue that will be biopsied. **B** Hold the needle still and advance the stylette into the tissue. Some of the tissue bulges against the thin shaft of the stylette **C** Hold the stylette still and advance the needle to cut off and enclose the core of tissue. **D** Withdraw the needle and retrieve the core of tissue.

needle into the lesion, hold the stylette still, withdraw then advance the needle to close it.

c. Draw out the closed needle, then retract the needle to expose the specimen resting on the thinned section of the stylette. Place the specimen in the appropriate fixative and immediately label the container, fill out the request form and ensure that the specimen is sent promptly to the laboratory.

4. A spring-loaded wide-bore needle can be used, or a drill biopsy – a high-speed rotating hollow needle.

5. All forms of needle biopsy may cause severe bleeding, so apply steady pressure over the track for 3–5 minutes timed by the clock.

OPEN BIOPSY

1. **Excision biopsy** implies removing the whole structure or lesion such as a discrete lump on its own or lying within more homogeneous tissue. This is intended to remove completely the lesion while providing material for histological examination.

2. **Incision biopsy** involves the removal of a portion from a large structure. It provides material for study but is not intended to remove the whole of the diseased tissue. Always try to include junctional tissue between diseased and normal tissues, where the architecture is recognizable. If an edge is present, excise a wedge from it, leaving a defect,

which can usually be closed with sutures (Fig. 7.3). If there is no edge, excise an ellipse in the shape of a boat with the keel lying in the depths (Fig. 7.4). If you need to biopsy a deeply placed lump, make sure you can reach it safely without injuring nearby structures. Be willing to make an adequate incision so you can identify structures you may encounter.

3. A **hooked wire marker** is used especially in the breast when a suspicious area such as a small mass or collection of microcalcification is identified on mammography or other imaging technique. As a rule the radiologist inserts a hollow needle into the suspicious area, introducing through this a hooked or curved wire before withdrawing the needle (Fig. 7.5). You should now approach the suspicious area by the most direct route. Cut through the outer part of the wire, leaving the hook marker in place. Excise the suspicious area and marker, if necessary X-raying the specimen to confirm that the correct tissue has been excised.

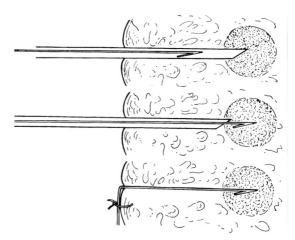

Fig. 7.5 The suspicious lesion has been identified by surface measurement, stereotactic measurement or ultrasound. After inserting a needle into it, pass through the needle a hooked or bent wire and then remove the needle. You may bend the wire and suture it flush with the skin to prevent it from being dislodged.

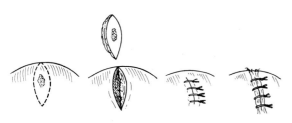

Fig. 7.3 Cut a wedge from the edge of a structure and appose the cut surfaces with stitches.

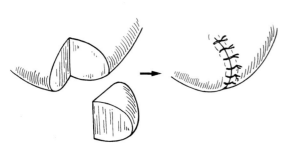

Fig. 7.4 Away from an edge, excise a boat-shaped specimen. If the tissue is supple you may be able to close the defect as a linear scar. If it is not, insert stitches and tie them, after drawing in nearby tissue to fill the defect, if possible. Alternatively, lay in gelatine foam or a similar haemostatic substance.

CONNECTIVE TISSUE

1. This varies from flimsy areolar tissue (L *areola*, diminutive of *area* = an open, empty place), to tough ligaments, tendons and aponeuroses (G *apo* = from + *neuron* = a nerve or tendon), which may be considered as flattened tendons attached to muscles. The vascularity of stable connective tissue is minimal but blood vessels may cross connective tissue spaces, bound for other tissues and organs.

2. Tendons and aponeuroses have most of the fibres running in one direction – along the line of the attached muscle contraction.

AREOLAR TISSUE

This occupies the space between structures that move relative to each other, for example between muscles, around tendons. It is an important guide to tissue planes and often has slack vessels crossing it to supply a moving structure.

1. Cut it with scalpel or scissors, preferably after sealing any fine vessels with diathermy. Occasionally, it can be gently stripped with your fingers.

2. Repair it using very fine absorbable stitches mounted on a round-bodied needle.

APONEUROSES

1. Because these transmit the pull of muscles, the fibres tend to run parallel, although cross-fibres bind the parallel fibres together. Whenever possible split the fibres; they need to be cut with a strong scalpel or scissors.

2. Repair aponeuroses with strong, synthetic absorbable or non-absorbable thread on round-bodied or trocar-pointed needles. When the cut is across the fibres, rejoin it using horizontal mattress sutures, since simple stitches tend to cut out if tension is exerted on them (Fig. 7.6). Conversely, if the cut is parallel to the majority of the fibres place the stitches at varying distances from the edges to prevent a strip from being detached (Fig. 7.7).

3. Healing of aponeuroses is slow. If they are subjected to strain at an early stage, the repair will give way or stretch. The ability to stretch is increased during pregnancy, in nutritional deficiency and in old age. In some diseases there are molecular defects in collagen or elastic fibres.

4. It may be necessary to bolster aponeurotic repairs. In the past, biological and artificial materials have been inserted, which worked by creating an inflammatory reaction that provoked the laying down of fibrous tissue. At present, non-absorbable synthetic meshes, usually of polypropylene or polyester, are used; they evoke little inflammatory reaction but are incorporated into the tissues. They are cut larger than the defect to overlap the edges and are sutured or stapled in place.

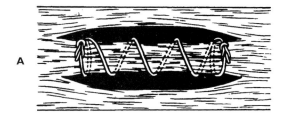

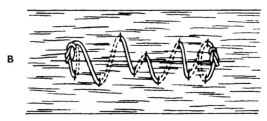

Fig. 7.7 The aponeurosis has been split between the fibres. **A** Stitches inserted all at the same distance from the edges tend to drag away a strip of fibres. **B** Stitches hold better if they are inserted at varying intervals from the edges.

TENDONS

1. These are composed of aligned collagen and elastic fibres to transmit the pull of muscles. If they are split in the line of the fibres they often eventually heal without loss of strength. If they are transected across the fibres, the ends retract. Following repair, the join is weak and stitches tend to cut out.

2. Stainless-steel sutures were previously used but synthetic polyamide, polyester or polypropylene have improved the results. The larger the area of the repair the greater the chance of a satisfactory repair; the ends may therefore be cut obliquely or stepwise.

3. Tendon repairs are often performed using a tourniquet to ensure that the field is not obscured with blood.

4. Be particularly careful where a close-fitting tendon changes direction over a fibro-osseus pulley-like smooth ridge or under an aponeurotic band, encased in a synovial sheath to reduce the friction. Do not injure the fine, mesentery-like connections bringing the blood supply from the deep surface, or the delicate mesothelial cells lining the synovium. If you leave an irregularity at such sites, adhesions develop between the tendon and the sheath, limiting or preventing movement.

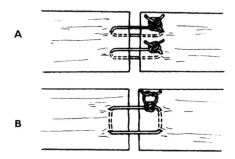

Fig. 7.6 The aponeurosis has been cut across the fibres. **A** Simple stitches tend to cut out. **B** Horizontal mattress sutures hold better.

5. Do not grasp the tendon ends with forceps; you will have a crushing effect and also damage and cause roughening of the surface; therefore, manipulate them with needles. One method is to transfix each of them with a straight needle about 2–2.5 cm from the cut ends. The needles can be drawn together and rotated as necessary, but protect the points to prevent needle-stick injury. Make sure that the clean-cut ends come together, if necessary by flexing the joint across which the tendon acts. The ends should fit together, without any twist, angulation or step.

6. Repair the tendon with a mattress stitch. Insert a stitch, usually of braided, synthetic polyester, into one end, emerging 1.5 cm from the end. Now reinsert the needle close to where it emerged, to cross the diameter of the tendon transversely, immediately opposite the point of insertion. Reinsert the needle close to the point of emergence, to emerge at the cut end. Bridge the gap between the cut ends and enter the other end, emerging 1.5 cm from the end, crossing the diameter of the tendon, back to the cut end (Fig. 7.8). It is often convenient to employ a straight needle but hold it with a needle-holder. Draw the two ends together, ensuring that they fit without twisting. Tie a perfect knot that will lie between the ends, holding the ends in perfect apposition, without bunching. Finally, insert a fine monofilament circumferential stitch to draw into continuity the paratenon, producing the smoothest possible surface.

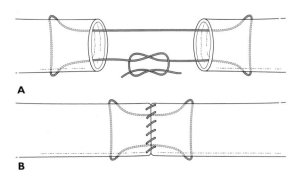

A

B

Fig. 7.8 Repair of a tendon. **A** Insert stitches bridging the tendons. Draw the ends together and tie a knot that will be buried between the apposed ends. **B** Insert very fine continuous stitches to repair the paratenon.

7. Following repair, reduce tension to a minimum by immobilizing joints in a position that brings the muscle origin and insertion as close as possible. Collagen laid down during healing stretches if it is strained so, unless the muscle pull is restrained, the tendon will be lengthened and subsequently the muscle action will be restricted.

LIGAMENTS

1. These are bands or sheets of fibrous tissue connecting bones, cartilages and other structures (L *ligare* = to bind or tie), or act as supports for fascia or muscles.

2. Torn supporting ligaments can often be repaired in a similar manner to aponeuroses or tendons.

3. Ligaments that stabilize joints such as the collateral and cruciate ligaments of the knee are challenging to repair and demand specialist expertise. Unless they retain their length and strength the joint becomes unstable. Some can be repaired like tendons. Cruciate ligaments can be repaired using the central portion of the patellar tendon with a piece of the tibia and the patella at each end, which can be anchored in tunnels within the femur and tibia.

4. Allografts (G *allos* = other) such as bovine collateral ligament have been used, and a number of artificial materials such as carbon fibre, polyester and polytetrafluoroethylene.

NERVES

- Nerve fibres are enclosed within and protected by an endoneural sheath, the perineurium encloses bundles or fasciculi, and around the whole nerve is the epineurium (Fig. 7.9).
- Neuropraxia (G *prassein* = to do) is a temporary physiological block; in axonotmesis (G *temnein* = to cut) the axon but not the endoneurium is disrupted. Wallerian degeneration (Augustus Waller 1816–1870, English physiologist), occurs in the distal axon. The proximal axon sprouts distally along the intact endoneural tube, eventually connecting with the end organ.

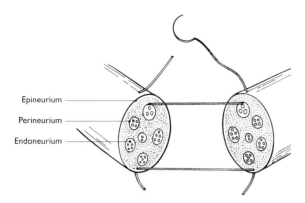

Epineurium ─────────

Perineurium ─────────

Endoneurium ─────────

Fig. 7.9   Repairing a cut nerve. Groups of fibres are encased in an endoneurial sheath, the fasciculi have a perineurium and the nerve has an epineurium. Ensure that the ends are brought into perfect alignment with the bundles correctly orientated, without tension or rotation. In some cases you need to use epineural stitches only, in others you can connect the perineurial sheaths.

- In neurotmesis the nerve is disrupted. If the nerve ends are coapted, axon sprouts enter the distal endoneurial tubes but the result is invariably less than perfect. Recovery of function is proportional to the perfection with which the original orientation is achieved, so that axons enter the correct distal endoneurial tubes.

   Key points

- The sooner you perform the repair and the more expertly you repair it, the better the result.
- You may first need to eliminate infection and bleeding, achieve skeletal stability, and assure primary skin closure.
- If you cannot fulfil these conditions, join the ends with a single stitch, close the skin or cover the nerve with well vascularized tissue, elevate the part to prevent oedema and delay repair until the conditions are suitable.

---

1. Ensure that there is adequate exposure, good light, available magnification with fine, micro-surgical instruments and a loupe or operating microscope (see Ch. 5, pp. 97–100).

2. If the nerve ends are ragged, trim them with a razor blade so you can appose them in perfect orientation.

3. Carefully unite the epineural sheaths using monofilament 8/0–10/0 nylon. In some cases, fascicular repair is possible.

4. If a segment of the nerve is lost, or the ends have retracted, you may interpose a graft, usually taken from the sural (L *sura* = calf of the leg) nerve. This does, however, prejudice the final result.

5. Following repair and closure, immobilize a limb in a position that avoids traction on the repair.

SKELETAL MUSCLE

1. Relaxed muscle is remarkably fragile and easily crushed. In contrast, healthy contracted muscle is remarkably resistant to injury.

2. If the motor nerve supply is lost the muscle is paralysed and atrophies (G *a* = not + *trephein* = to feed).

3. If a muscle is transected the muscle fibres do not reunite, but they are connected by intervening fibrosis. The single muscle becomes double-bellied.

4. If muscle is ischaemic as a result of loss of blood supply or constriction, it atrophies and is replaced with fibrous tissue; as this matures it contracts, causing contractures described in 1872 by the German surgeon Richard Volkmann.

5. Since muscle fibres run parallel to each other, if they are separated they can be re-apposed using absorbable sutures mounted on round-bodied needles, but do not tie the sutures tightly or they will strangulate the muscle fibres and cut out. If muscles are cut across the fibres, the ends contract and become distracted. Stitches inserted to re-appose the ends tend to cut out unless you use horizontal mattress sutures, but try to minimize tension by bringing the origin and insertion as close together as possible until the repair is sound.

6. Avoid muscle ischaemia from too tight application of encircling plasters. If the distal circulation is prejudiced, split the plaster longitudinally. If muscle swells within tight fascia or skin, following,

for example, an encircling burn, split the skin and fascia longitudinally; this is the original meaning of 'debride' (F = unbridle, release).

CARTILAGE

1. Pure cartilage covers the ends of bones in contact at joints, or as menisci is interposed between bone ends. Its has limited ability to regenerate dependent upon its blood supply, usually from the peripheral attachments. It usually heals with deposition of fibrocartilage.

2. Fibrocartilage can be cut and sutured and stitched after drilling stitch holes, and can be transplanted from one site to another as part of a composite graft.

MUCOPERIOSTEUM

This is a strong conjoint double layer with a good blood supply, covering among other areas the hard palate and bony nasal walls.

1. Choose the suture material depending on the feasibility of removing the stitches. If they can be removed, 3/0 black silk, which is easy to see, or monofilament nylon, which evokes minimal reaction, may be appropriate, mounted on half-curved, reverse-cutting, eyeless needles.

2. If it is difficult or impossible to remove stitches, insert 4/0 synthetic absorbable stitches.

SOFT TISSUES

BREAST

- When operating on the breast constantly remember the radial distribution of the lobules, which drain centrally to reach the nipple.
- Cysts can be aspirated and the fluid sent for cytological examination. During lactation, retained milk may produce galactoceles (G *galaktos* = milk + *kele* = a swelling) and infection of the breast can result in abscess formation.
- Palpable lumps can be investigated with fine-needle aspiration cytology, needle biopsy or open biopsy.
- Impalpable lumps detected by imaging can be marked with a hooked wire so that they can be identified during biopsy (see p. 118).

1. Plan incisions to take into account the cosmetic result. Skin tension lines are mainly transverse before the breast develops but as it fills and eventually sags they change. Circumareolar incisions give a good cosmetic result but remember that they may transect the lactiferous ducts.

2. A consideration when making incisions for biopsy is the importance of the possible need to incorporate it in a mastectomy incision if this becomes necessary.

3. When removing a biopsy specimen avoid damaging the architecture. Hold on to attached connective tissue, not the lump itself.

4. Avoid the development of a haematoma by achieving perfect haemostasis and apposing the cut edges of breast tissue with fine absorbable synthetic sutures. A suction drain may help (see Ch. 11, p. 163).

5. Close the skin to produce the best possible cosmetic result.

LYMPH NODES

- Enlargement of lymph nodes indicates local inflammation, infection or other disease; alternatively it may be a local manifestation of generalized disease.
- Enlarged nodes may be singular, multiple, discrete, matted, mobile or fixed. Superficial enlarged nodes are usually palpable although the physical signs may be misleading. Deeply placed nodes can be demonstrated by various methods of imaging, or displayed at operation.
- Before operation discuss with the pathologist how to prepare the specimen, and which receptacles are needed.

1. Carry out fine-needle aspiration cytology and needle biopsy only if you are confident of the anatomy; otherwise, recruit the aid of a radiologist, who can use ultrasound or other imaging methods for guidance.

2. Lymph nodes are fragile and if they are crushed the accuracy of the diagnosis is prejudiced.

Chapter 7: Handling connective and soft tissues

> ## Key point
>
> - Lymph node biopsy is not a minor or casual procedure; most nodes are in close proximity to important structures. Never attempt to remove a node without studying the anatomy and obtaining adequate exposure. Many surgical disasters result from a cavalier attitude to removing what appears to be a solitary, mobile lymph node.

3. Place the incision in a skin crease if possible and approach the node with caution. Lymph nodes may be very fragile, especially if they are diseased. Having reached the surface of the node, work around the sides but do not grasp it with forceps because you may damage it; if possible leave a little connective tissue attached to it so that you can grasp this.

4. As you reach the deeper aspects, move the mobilized gland from side to side so that you can examine its attachments from different aspects. Remember that the vessels usually enter from the undersurface and that there may be an adherent important structure. The majority of complications arise because we are tempted to lift the gland, put the resulting pedicle under tension, cut it – and often regret it.

5. Carefully check the field and ensure total haemostasis.

6. On occasion, you must remove one or a few glands from a matted mass. Do not damage glands you do not intend to remove.

7. Divide up the node, without crushing it, into the required number of specimens and place them in the appropriate receptacles.

8. Close the wound to give the best possible cosmetic result.

ABDOMINAL WALL

1. Never forget that the usual purpose of incisions in the abdomen is to achieve the best possible access to structures within the cavity.

2. Whenever possible, avoid cutting through muscle. This can be achieved in two standard incisions, a midline vertical and a 'gridiron' incision for appendicectomy.

3. I shall describe the technique for a right-handed surgeon. You may need to reverse some of the instructions if you are left-handed.

Midline abdominal incision

As a rule you stand on the supine patient's right side.

1. The midline abdominal incision divides the skin, linea alba and peritoneum. It can be in the upper or lower abdomen, or central, by skirting the umbilicus. Divide the skin with the belly of the scalpel, holding the knife so that it cuts vertically. Start at the upper end, cutting from your left to right.

2. After achieving haemostasis, continue in the same line through the white, firm, fibrous linea alba and then stop as you reach a variable layer of fat overlying the fused fascia transversalis and peritoneum.

3. Pick up the final layer with the tips of a haemostat to tent it, allowing you to grasp it again, alongside the first grip. Remove and then replace the first forceps while holding up the peritoneum with the second forceps, in case you had initially and inadvertently picked up an abdominal viscus. Now have both haemostats held up, tenting the peritoneum while you make a small incision between them. This allows air to enter the abdomen so that viscera can fall clear (Fig. 7.10). Insert a finger into the peritoneal cavity and move it in a complete circle to confirm that there is no viscus in danger. Having assured yourself, insert one blade of Mayo's scissors and carefully slit the peritoneum in the line of the initial incision.

4. To close the incision, grasp the peritoneum at each end with strong, straight haemostatic forceps and have them lifted clear of the underlying viscera by your assistant. Your may also apply similar forceps in the middle of each edge, allowing the handles to lie outwards, everting the edges. Take a round-bodied, curved, sharp or blunt taper-pointed needle (see p. 36), with a non-absorbable suture such as 1.0 monofilament nylon four times the wound length.

5. It is usually most convenient to suture from the upper end to the lower end – from your non-dominant to your dominant side, as the incision lies transversely in front of you. Take a bite through all

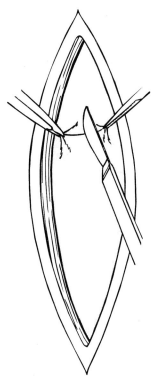

Fig. 7.10 Incising the peritoneum after tenting it between two forceps.

layers, except the skin and subcutaneous tissues, from out to in on the far side, in to out on the near side, and tie the suture securely. Ensure that the bristly short end is well buried. Alternatively you may use a thinner suture that has both ends inserted into the needle, forming a closed loop. Insert your first stitch, then pass the needle through the loop – this produces a less bulky means of securing the start of the suture line.

6. Now insert a continuous, over-and-over stitch until you reach the other end. Drive the needle from without in on the far side, from within out on the near side, approximately every 1 cm, placed 1 cm from the edge.

7. Carefully avoid overtightening the stitches. Once you have apposed the edges, have your assistant steady the emerging thread so you can avoid the sawing action of tightening, slackening and re-tightening the stitches.

8. Take care to avoid injuring structures with the

last few stitches by inserting them slackly, with the edges separated, then tightening them seriatim.

9. At the end, hold on to the final loop on one side and the single thread on the other. You may either tie the loop to the single thread or employ an Aberdeen knot (see Ch. 3, p. 42). As a rule, do not insert subcutaneous stitches.

10. Now carefully close the skin with interrupted or continuous stitches.

 Key point

- Ceaselessly and vigilantly protect the abdominal contents from injury. Place every stitch carefully, through all the intended layers. Do not damage the suture material or you will weaken it. Overtightened stitches strangulate the tissues and are likely to cut out, risking burst abdomen. Tie knots securely and turn the bristly ends under, so they do not project under the skin.

Gridiron incision

1. The incision is named after the crossed iron bars laid over a fire on which to grill food, which resemble the crossed muscle layers. It is associated with the New York surgeon Charles McBurney (1845–1913), who established the diagnosis and surgical treatment of appendicitis. He described a point in the right iliac fossa at the junction of the middle and outer thirds of a line between the umbilicus and anterior superior iliac spine where the maximal tenderness is felt in the disease and on which the incision is centred.

2. Make the skin incision centred on the point but in the line of skin tension – described by Otto Lanz of Amsterdam (1865–1935) – and incise the subcutaneous tissue in the same line.

3. You expose the shining aponeurosis of external oblique muscle. Split the fibres without cutting them, to reveal the fibres of internal oblique muscle, at right angles to the external oblique, and split these to reveal the fibres of transversus abdominis muscle. For each layer, make a small incision with a scalpel, then gently insert the tips of Mayo's scissors into the

gap and open them in the line of the fibres. Split these to reveal the conjoint transversalis fascia and peritoneum (Fig. 7.11).

4. Pick up the peritoneum with artery forceps to tent it, grasp the raised tented portion, release and regrasp the peritoneum with the first forceps. Have the two forceps held up while you make a small scalpel incision between them, to let in air and allow the viscera to fall away. Insert a finger to ensure that there is no adherent structure before introducing one blade of a pair of scissors to enlarge the opening fully within the muscle boundaries.

5. Close the incision in layers. First, hold up the ends of the peritoneal incision and insert a continuous suture of 2/0 or 3/0 absorbable synthetic suture to close it, ensuring that you do not injure any intra-abdominal structure. Using the same material, insert interrupted stitches to appose each of the muscle layers, taking care not to pull the stitches tight. Finally, close the skin using interrupted or continuous sutures. To achieve a good cosmetic result you might wish to insert a subcuticular stitch (see Ch. 3, pp. 105–106).

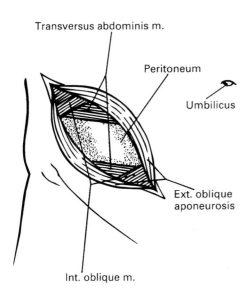

Fig. 7.11 The gridiron incision for appendicectomy. Split but do not cut the fibres of the aponeurosis and muscles to reach the peritoneum.

ORGANS

BOWEL

1. Provided the normally rich blood supply is intact and edges are carefully apposed, bowel (L *botellus* = a sausage) heals well (see Ch. 4).

2. Although the contents of the small bowel are normally almost sterile, as soon as there is any stagnation following an injury, micro-organisms flourish here, as they normally do in the colon.

Key point

- Repaired bowel must have: a good blood supply, perfect apposition of the edges, absence of tension.

LIVER

Liver is amenable to fine-needle aspiration or to needle biopsy. Ultrasound or other imaging methods may be used to guide the needle to lesions. A fine needle can be inserted percutaneously into the intra-hepatic bile ducts and contrast media injected into them to produce a cholangiogram (G *chole* = bile + *angeion* = vessel + *graphein* = to write).

1. Liver is honeycombed with blood vessels and bile ducts so that it bleeds and oozes bile when cut. At operation on the liver, control bleeding and bile leakage using diathermy current and employing blunt dissection. 'Finger fracture' consists of compressing a portion of liver between finger and thumb, destroying the liver cells but not dividing the vessels and ducts; these can be identified, doubly ligated and divided. Ultrasound tissue disruption achieves a similar purpose. The vessels and ducts can be identified, doubly ligated and divided.

2. After achieving haemostasis, insert absorbable synthetic sutures mounted on large, round-bodied, curved needles to appose the cut surfaces whenever possible. Take bites well away from the cut edges and do not tie them too tightly or they will cut out. In some cases it is beneficial to insert stitches parallel with the edges to slightly constrict and

support them before placing stitches to appose the cut edges (Fig. 7.12).

3. A variety of haemostatic materials can be applied

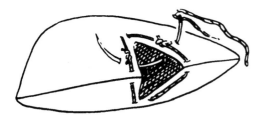

Fig. 7.12 Suture the liver using a large, round-bodied needle. It may be an advantage to insert an encircling stitch close to the edges before bringing the edges together with apposing stitches placed outside these.

SPLEEN

In the past splenectomy was carried out with little concern as part of other procedures, if it was even slightly damaged. The dangers of post-splenectomy infection are now recognized, so that it is preserved whenever possible. The former aggressive attitude stemmed from the propensity of the damaged spleen to continue to bleed or develop recurrent bleeding.

1. A capsular tear may seal if you apply haemostatic agents such as fibrin glue, gelatin sponge, polyglycolic mesh, microfibrillar collagen or crushed muscle.

2. If there is a tear into the pulp, consider inserting stitches to close it, if necessary tying the stitches over gelatin sponge or a tongue of omentum.

3. If you need to remove the spleen, consider placing slices of it into pockets constructed in the greater omentum.

4. Determine to give antipneumococcal vaccine postoperatively. Advise adults to seek treatment at the first sign of infection and give children prophylactic penicillin for 2 years.

PANCREAS

The pancreas (G *pan* = all + *kreas* = flesh) is well protected from injury but is very fragile. If the

enzymes are released and activated they are extremely erosive.

1. The gland does not hold stitches well, so repair is difficult to achieve.

2. The body or the tail can be removed, followed by closure of the main duct.

3. Close the parenchyma (G *para* = beside + *encheo* = to pour in. The substance of the organ; from the ancient belief that it was poured in and then congealed). The closure is best achieved by cutting the stump in the shape of a fishtail (Fig. 7.13), then suturing the edges.

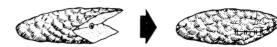

Fig. 7.13 Repairing the pancreas. Cut the stump end like a fish tail and suture together the two flaps you have created.

KIDNEY

This has a rich blood supply and a firm capsule that holds stitches well, and is amenable to repair provided the drainage system is intact.

URETER

This must be sutured with fine stitches to avoid obstructing the narrow channel (see Ch. 4, p. 74). If it must be repaired in the lower part, it may be preferable to join it directly to the bladder by raising a flap of bladder roof, formed into a tube to bridge the gap, associated with the name of Boari.

BLADDER

The wall is robust and holds sutures well. Many urologists exclude the lining epithelium from the stitches, which catch all the other layers.

UTERUS

The thick muscle is tough and holds stitches well. However the suture line leaves a scar that is relatively weak compared with the remainder of the wall. The uterine tubes have a narrow lumen. If they are to be repaired, use the finest sutures, inserted with great care, preferably under magnification (see Ch.5, pp. 97–100).

LUNG

The lung remains expanded because it fills the intermittently subatmospheric pleural cavity. It collapses if air enters the potential space, either through a breach in the chest wall or through a damaged lung.

1. A leak usually reseals if you insert a chest drain connected to an underwater seal (see Ch. 11, pp. 165–166).

2. Suture large tears in the lung using absorbable synthetic sutures.

HEART

Heart muscle holds stitches well and they can be inserted while the heart continues to beat. It is possible to stop the heart and bypass its pump action in order to perform delicate procedures on it or within the lumen.

ENDOCRINE AND OTHER GLANDS

Glandular tissue is relatively soft but the connective tissue usually provides good support. The thyroid gland is vascular, especially in thyrotoxic states. The adrenal gland is fragile and has small veins that are easily torn.

BRAIN AND SPINAL CORD

These are almost fluid, behaving somewhat like blancmange. If they are damaged, healing is by the deposition of connective glial tissue. The unmyelinated nerve fibres cannot easily reconnect.

1. Nerve tracts can be divided within the brain and in the spinal cord by direct approach or by stereotactic (*stereos* = solid, three dimensional + *tassein* = to arrange) techniques.

2. The brain is richly supplied with blood vessels, which may become blocked or bleed. These may be treatable by interventional radiographic techniques.

8

Handling bone

with Deborah Eastwood

Exposure
Steadying
Biopsy
Cutting
Drilling
Screws
Stitching
Wiring
Plates
External fixators
Intramedullary fixation
Bone grafts
Amputation
Joints

- Techniques and tools for operating on bone have been mainly adapted from carpentry, masonry and engineering.
- Wood and metal are relatively homogeneous; bone is not. Cortical bone is thick and dense in young adults, thin and less dense in the elderly. Bone strength and density are affected by disease.
- Bone infection does not respond well to antibiotics and tends to become chronic. Avoid the risk of contamination of the patient and yourself by using instruments to manipulate bone when possible, wearing two pairs of gloves and handling the bone as little as possible.
- Bony union occurs only if the surfaces are brought into contact. Perfect apposition, absence of movement and compression of the fragments achieves primary union. A haematoma develops if there is movement or separation of the fragments; this is invaded in turn by granulation tissue, cartilage and osteoid tissue, called 'callus', which later ossifies.
- Rigid fixation allows early return of function and

weight bearing, avoiding joint stiffness and muscle wasting.

EXPOSURE

1. Revise the anatomy of the approach to avoid damaging overlying structures. Many approaches are standardized – learn and apply them.

2. Do not excessively strip or destroy the periosteum since it carries the nutrient blood vessels and the deep layer is rich in osteoblasts.

STEADYING

1. Do not work on unfixed and unsteadied bone with sharp tools. Your tools will inevitably slip and damage the bone and vital soft tissues.

2. Make use of retractors, levers, forceps, guard plates, swabs and your assistants to protect the tissues from inadvertent damage (Fig. 8.1).

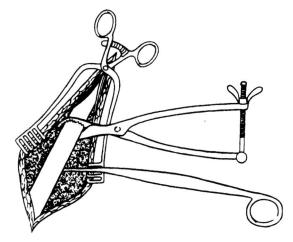

Fig. 8.1 Use a self-retaining retractor and a bone lever to expose a long bone. Have your assistant steady the bone with bone-holding forceps.

3. If you change your point of attack, reassess your safeguards and, if necessary, rearrange them.

BIOPSY

1. Although imaging methods have developed, histological diagnosis may still be required to elucidate general and bone disease.

2. If the area is soft, diagnostic cells can be recovered using fine-needle aspiration cytology, Tru-Cut® or drill biopsy (see Ch. 7, pp. 116–118). You may use imaging methods to guide the needle.

3. You may be able to obtain a specimen under local anaesthesia, with sedation if necessary, using a Jamishidi needle, which has a cross-piece by which it can be rotated with a trephining action.

4. You may be able to obtain a specimen of bone marrow using a trephine inserted through a small incision; this cuts a cylinder of cortex and underlying marrow.

5. Open biopsy, usually under general anaesthesia, requires exposure of the bone. Use cutting tools to remove bone; soft tissues can be removed with a knife or curette.

CUTTING

Hand saw

1. Hand saws are infrequently used except for major amputations.

2. Decide the line of the cut and expose it fully, clear of other structures.

3. Protect the soft tissues in the line of the cut and those that might be damaged if the saw blade slips.

4. Hand saws are designed to make straight cuts. Do not attempt to change the line of the cut or you risk jamming the blade. Start a fresh line.

5. Start the cut by drawing the blade towards you, steadying it against your non-dominant thumb, placed well above the teeth (Fig. 8.2).

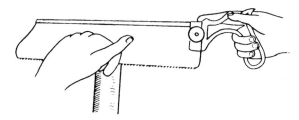

Fig. 8.2   Start the saw cut by drawing the blade towards you, steadying the blade with the non-dominant thumb placed high up on the blade.

6. In some cases you can use a saw guide.

7. Use a steady, rhythmic, to-and-fro movement, the full length of the blade, putting no downward pressure on the saw.

8. At the end of the cut avoid putting a strain on the bone or you will fracture it. Prefer to lighten the movement so that the last section does not suddenly give way. In some cases you can make a counter-cut from the opposite side so the break occurs away from the edge and avoids leaving a sharp projecting splinter.

Powered saws

1. Most saws are now powered. Circular rotation is potentially dangerous because the unengaged portion of the blade is liable to damage other tissues – or you. A reciprocating saw (L *re* = backwards + *pro* = forwards) is less dangerous (Fig. 8.3).

2. Radially oscillating (L *oscillare* + to swing) blades, sawing in a segment of a circle only (Fig. 8.4), reduce the cutting area.

3. The saw blade heats up during long cuts. In order to avoid overheating the bone, cool the blade with saline.

4. Do not use blunt blades in powered saws – they cut unreliably.

 Key point

- Remember that saws remove a wider thickness of bone than the thickness of the blade, because of the 'set' of the teeth.

 Key point

- Be doubly careful when nearing the end of the cut in case the saw rapidly over-runs the desired course

---

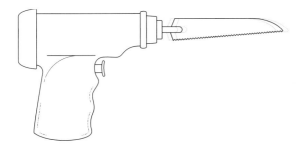

Fig. 8.3 The powered reciprocating saw moves back and forth in the same manner as a hand saw.

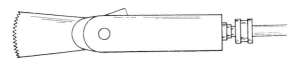

Fig. 8.4 This powered oscillating saw blade moves in a limited segment of a circle.

Chisel

1. A chisel (OF *cisel*, from L *caedere* = to cut) is distinguished by having a bevel on one side (Fig. 8.5), so that it resists cutting along a straight path. Wood chisels are often pushed by hand but a bone chisel needs to be driven by a mallet; in consequence it is made robust, relatively thick and acts, when driven into bone, as a powerful wedge.

2. If you place the chisel on a bony surface, bevel uppermost and tap it, it may chip off a flake of superficial bone. As it bites further in, the bevel makes it angle deeper so that the handle swings more vertically. There is a danger that, because of the thickness of the chisel, it will fracture the bone (Fig. 8.6).

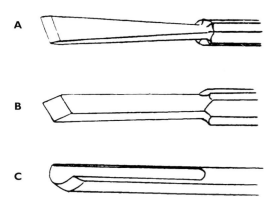

Fig. 8.5 A Osteotome. **B** Chisel. **C** Gouge.

3. If the bevel is on the undersurface, you need to start the cut with the tool held more vertically or it will fail to bite, and will slide along the surface. As soon as the bevel enters the bone, the chisel tends to lift the edge on the unbevelled side and the handle is angled downwards. When you drive the chisel further, the effect of the bevel is to guide the cutting edge towards the surface, lifting off a sliver (OE *slifan* = to cleave) of superficial bone, as the chisel lies almost parallel with the surface.

4. A gouge (Fig. 8.5), has a hollow blade to scoop out. The bevel is on the outside so that it does not bite deeply.

Osteotome

1. This has bevels on both sides and can be thin because it is designed to make only straight cuts (Fig. 8.5).

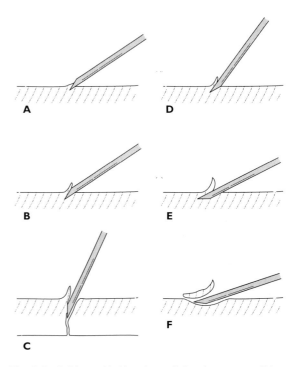

Fig. 8.6 Driving a chisel into bone. **A** Bevel uppermost. **B** It tends to angle vertically as it bites more deeply. **C** It becomes even more vertical and may split the bone. **D** Bevel on the underside. **E** The chisel tip lifts a sliver of bone and tends to flatten. **F** The chisel has cut out and lies almost parallel with the bone surface.

2. Plan the cut carefully to avoid deviation, which would strain the thin metal shaft.

3. To prevent shattering the sometimes brittle cortical bone, either first drill holes in the line of the cut or cut chips out of the cortex at the beginning to allow it to accommodate the thickness of the blade (Fig. 8.7).

4. Hold the osteotome or chisel in your non-dominant hand and drive it using a mallet (Fig. 8.8). Note the short handle of the mallet – an indication that you must not use too great force.

> ### Key point
>
> - Steady the hand holding the osteotome or chisel in such a way that you prevent the tool from slipping to one side or cutting through the bone into the soft tissues beyond.

Cutting forceps

1. These act like scissors (Fig. 8.9) so that you can make small cuts through bone that is not too thick or brittle, such as a rib, although a special guillotine-type tool is available for this purpose.

2. This tool inevitably has a crushing effect on the bone. In case of doubt, therefore, prefer to use a saw when this is appropriate.

Rongeurs

1. There are several versions of these (Fig. 8.9) and, as the name implies (F *ronger* = to gnaw), they nibble away bone.

2. They are valuable for shaping or excising bone from difficult corners or bony cavities.

3. Rongeurs are useful for obtaining specimens for histology from bone or other hard tissues. Because the jaws are hollowed out, they do not

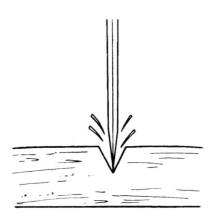

Fig. 8.7 Widen the cut as the osteotome bites deeper by successively chipping flakes from each side so that the thickness of the instrument can be accommodated to prevent splitting.

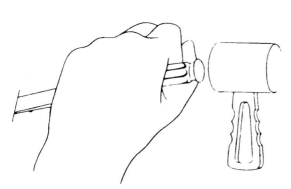

Fig. 8.8 Cutting with an osteotome or chisel. Steady the hand holding the tool to prevent it from slipping to one side or cutting right through the bone and damaging soft tissues beyond.

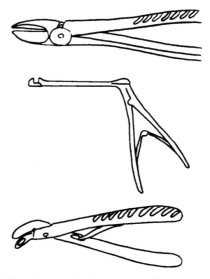

Fig. 8.9 Bone-cutting forceps at top. Rongeurs at centre and bottom; these have cupped blades so fragments of detached bone are grasped but not crushed, and can be removed.

excessively crush and destroy the architecture of the specimens.

File

Because bone is not homogeneous like metal and wood, files tend to be used only for rasping sharp edges from angular cuts made with saws and other instruments, as following an amputation.

DRILLING

1. Hand drills (Fig. 8.10) are not now used routinely for drilling bone. It may be difficult to start the hole, especially on rounded, hard, cortical bone, without first making a preliminary notch with an awl or sharp punch. The drill point often tends to 'walk' away from the intended point of penetration.

2. Because two hands are fully occupied with holding and turning the drill, it is difficult to control. It may be important to limit the penetration of the bit (the boring piece). In such circumstances, take precautions to prevent this, for example by ensuring that only the required length of the bit protrudes from the chuck or by fixing a clamp to the bit that acts as a buffer when it hits the bone surface.

3. A hand brace can be used as when trephining the skull (Fig. 8.11); in this case the bit is not a drill but a shaped, cutting perforator that prevents sudden uncontrolled penetration. The opening in the skull can then be enlarged using burrs, which act like circular files.

4. Powered drills (Fig. 8.12) are now routinely employed. Properly controlled, they allow you to concentrate on the process of drilling, since you do not have to turn the bit yourself. However, since they rotate at a higher speed than manual drills, they may easily 'run away'. Identify and carefully protect vulnerable soft tissues. Powered drills create heat; cool the bit with cold, sterile, physiological saline and avoid long periods of continuous drilling.

5. Once a hole is drilled it may be enlarged using a reamer. Various shaping bits can be used, as when preparing a joint socket for replacement.

6. The availability of accurately made prostheses (G *pros* = to + *thesis* = a putting; hence an addition or substitution, for example for lost parts), demands that they are accurately fitted. When you intend to fix bones by screwing on metal plates and similar devices, you must drill the holes accurately both for perfect alignment and also to ensure that the bone is not excessively weakened. Whenever possible make use of drill guides (Fig. 8.13). For many standardized procedures special drill guides form part of the kit to enable you to drill screw holes accurately.

7. Clear away bone chips after drilling a hole.

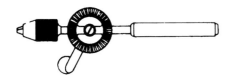

Fig. 8.10　Hand drill.

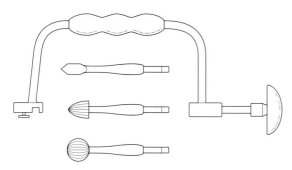

Fig. 8.11　Brace and tools for opening the skull. At the top is a perforator and below are two types of burr.

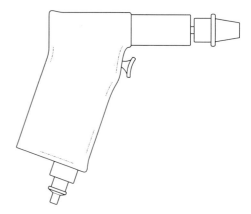

Fig. 8.12　Powered drill.

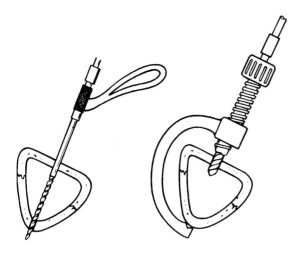

Fig. 8.13 Drill guides. The one on the left is hand held; the one on the right can be firmly attached to the bone, leaving you two hands to control the drill.

 Key points

- Control drills.
- Constantly check that the exit is free from tissues that could be damaged.
- Do not angle drills – the bits are brittle and will break.
- Do not exert excessive pressure or you will jam the bit.
- Avoid catching up soft tissues and swabs in the rotating bit

SCREWS

1. Properly used, screws are very versatile and provide a valuable method of fixing bones, and of fixing plates and prostheses to bone.

2. They are made from a variety of metals, including stainless steel, vitallium and titanium. Pure titanium provokes almost no tissue reaction and also does not interfere with magnetic resonance imaging.

3. When using metals, ensure that they are compatible. If screws of one metal hold plates of another metal they generate electrolytic action, weakening the metal and provoking bone absorption.

4. Formerly, most screws were self-tapping – they cut a spiral channel to accommodate their screw-thread as they are inserted. Although self-tapping screws are still sometimes used, they do not have as strong a grip as screws inserted into pre-tapped holes (Fig. 8.14).

 Key point

- Do not screw cortical bone as you screw wood. Wood accepts the extra volume of a screw by compacting. Cortical bone is already compact and is brittle. Unless you provide an adequate hole, it will split. Cancellous bone behaves more like wood and can compact to accept screws.

5. When fixing long bones, use screws that pierce and grip both cortices, since these are the most compact and strong. For the best results, first drill a hole with a drill the same size as the shank of the screw, from which the thread flanges project. Measure the length of the hole so you can select the correct length of screw. Now use a tap of the correct size to cut the thread. Unscrew the tap, remove the loose bony fragments and insert the screw. This is illustrated in Figure 8.15.

6. Cortical screws are fully threaded (Fig. 8.16). If they are inserted and tightened through a fully tapped hole across a fracture with separation of the fracture surfaces, they do not exert any compression, since they merely hold the fragments in the same position

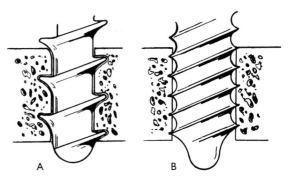

A   B

Fig. 8.14 A screw in a pre-tapped hole (**A**) has a much better grip than does a self-tapping screw (**B**).

Fig. 8.15 From top to bottom: drill a hole through both cortices; use a depth gauge to measure the required length of screw; tap the hole to cut the screw thread; insert and drive home the screw.

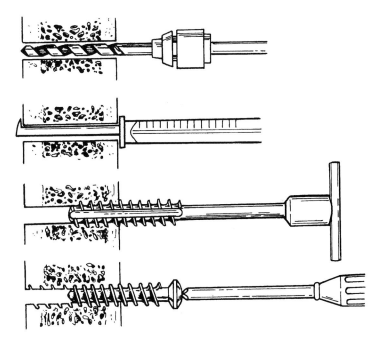

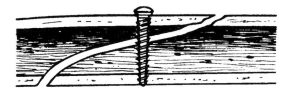

Fig. 8.16 A fully threaded screw inserted in a fully tapped track created while the bones remain apart will have no compression effect on the gap.

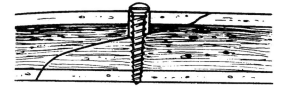

Fig. 8.17 If the proximal cortex is drilled oversize, the screw acts as a lag screw, compressing the bones.

in which they were tapped. If the proximal fragment is drilled oversized, the thread grips only in the distal fragment and exerts a compression effect (Fig. 8.17).

7. A cancellous screw, having part of the shaft unthreaded beneath the head (Fig. 8.18), does not require to have the proximal fragment drilled oversize but the screw does not grip the far cortex so do not use it.

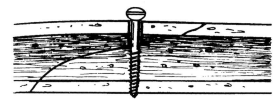

Fig. 8.18 Do not use a cancellous screw, with an unthreaded part of the shank, as an alternative to drilling the proximal fragment oversized and using a cortical screw. The cancellous screw will not grip the far cortex.

 Key point

- Do not overtighten screws; if you do you will strip the threads. Perform the final tightening with finger and thumb pressure on the screwdriver.

8. If you place a screw at right angles to unite oblique surfaces in a long bone, such as a fracture line, it will slip when longitudinal stresses are applied (Fig. 8.19). Instead, insert the screw perpendicular to the bone surface.

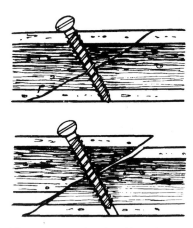

Fig. 8.19 The screw placed at right angles to an oblique fracture line allows movement when longitudinal stress is applied.

9. If there is a spiral fracture, insert the screws through the middle of the fragments along the bone, so they also form a spiral (Fig. 8.20).

10. If a screw-head protrudes and will interfere with function, cause pain or be unsightly, use a countersink drill bit to create a depression into which the screw head fits.

11. Sometimes retained screws and other metal inserts, such as plates, cause problems after they have served their purpose and may need to be removed. Biodegradable screws of polydioxanone, polylactic acid or polyglycolic:polylactic acid co-polymer are under trial.

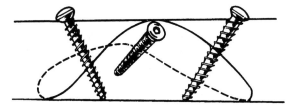

Fig. 8.20 Insert screws through the middle of the fragments to stabilize a spiral fracture, so they also form a spiral.

STITCHING

Stitches can be inserted into periosteum or ligaments. Alternatively, you may drill holes into which you can insert stitches. Special small screws can be inserted into bone that carry a thread. A similar screw can be inserted into another bone and the threads can then be tied together to join the bones.

WIRING

1. Bone can be fixed by encircling it with wire (Fig. 8.21). Encircling wire may prejudice the blood supply to the bone, so the method is used less often than formerly, and often the wire is removed later when it has served its purpose.

2. Twist the wire ends evenly. If you keep one end straight and wrap the other around it, it has no holding power. If you overtighten the wire, it will fracture. Turn the ends of the twisted wire so they do not protrude under the skin or press upon vulnerable structures.

3. As an alternative to encircling wire, drill holes through the bone and use wire like a stitch.

4. In some situations the bone can be stapled, especially if it is cancellous. Tap in the staple in an introducer, then remove the introducer so the staple can be driven fully home.

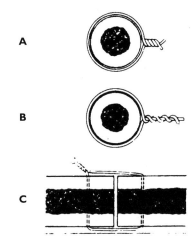

Fig. 8.21 Wiring bone. **A** The ends of the encircling wire are evenly twisted. **B** One wire has been wound round the other wire, which is straight. This is insecure. **C** Drill the bone and pass wire through the holes in the manner of a stitch.

PLATES

1. Metal plates are manufactured of stainless steel, vitallium and titanium (Fig. 8.22). They may be straight, angled, flat, tubular, with round or oval

holes, and with holes arranged in rows or staggered.

2. Plates may be used as struts to produce mechanical support, or as buttresses pushing in a fragment (Fig. 8.23)

3. At operation place the bones in correct alignment, select a suitable-sized plate and, if necessary, bend it to fit accurately. Make sure that at least three holes lie over each fragment.

4. Clamp the plate in place while drilling though the centre of each hole towards the opposite cortex, using a drill guide. Be very careful not to splinter the bone or damage soft tissues as the drill emerges at the opposite cortex. Estimate the required screw lengths using a depth gauge. Tap the holes and insert the screws (Fig. 8.24). Do not overtighten them.

5. Compressing the separated ends of the bone facilitates union. A simple method of achieving this is to use compression plates with longitudinally oriented oval holes. As the round-headed screw is tightened into the hole it distracts the plate, effectively shortening it (Fig. 8.25). If the other end of the plate has been firmly fixed to the other fragment, the result is to draw the bones together.

6. A special compression plate can be used. First, securely anchor one end on one side of the break. Apply the other component, crossing over the break (Fig. 8.26), so that the hook on the fully opened anchored section can engage in the nearest screw-hole. Fix the second plate at its far end from the compression device. Now tighten the screw to draw the two parts together. Insert intermediate screws on both sides of the break. Finally, release the compression device, unscrew it and insert the final screw in the plate that had been engaged with the compression device hook.

EXTERNAL FIXATORS

Many of these are complex and require advanced skills in order to employ them. Consequently they are described only to outline the principles on which they work. An important advantage is that the site of a break in continuity can be left undisturbed, fixation being undertaken at a distance on each side.

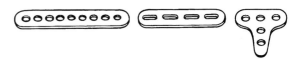
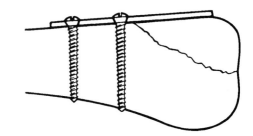

Fig. 8.22 Various metal plates.

Fig. 8.23 Plate used as a buttress to hold a fragment in place.

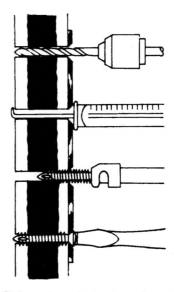

Fig. 8.24 Plating and screwing long bone. Ensure that the plate lies in contact along its length. From top to bottom: drill a hole through both cortices; measure the required screw length using a depth gauge; tap the hole; insert the screw, which should grip the opposite cortex as well as the near one.

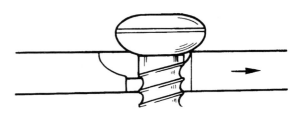

Fig. 8.25 As the round-headed screw-head is tightened into the oval hole in the plate, it produces distraction.

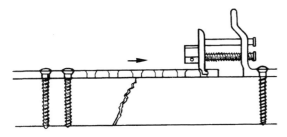

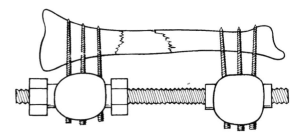

Fig. 8.26 Compression plate. Firmly fix the compression device on the right. Place the plate, crossing the break, so the hook on the fully opened compression device fits into the last screw hole. Fix the opposite end of the plate. Tighten the compression device. Place intermediate screws on both sides of the break. Slacken off and remove the compression device before inserting the last screw in the hole formerly occupied by the hook of the compression device.

Fig. 8.27 An external fixator.

1. Two or more threaded pins are inserted percutaneously, through small local incisions, into the bone on either side of the break, and at a distance from it. The pins can then be fixed with clamps at each site. After ensuring, usually with radiological confirmation, that the fragments are perfectly aligned, the clamps are locked on to a common external linkage (Fig. 8.27). The fixators can be adjusted and then relocked if necessary, and the distance between the two groups of fixing pins can be reduced or increased to compress or distract the ends. In some cases the pins are passed right through the limb and the projecting ends are attached to locking devices joined by a further linking device, so there is one on each side.

2. During the 1950s, G.A. Ilizarov in Kurgan, Siberia, developed a system of transfixing the bones above and below a break, using wires tensioned across external metal rings. The rings are linked across the break by rods and can be adjusted to compress or distract the ends (Fig. 8.28).

INTRAMEDULLARY FIXATION

1. Smooth, double-pointed wires of various lengths and diameters were invented by Martin Kirschner, Professor of Surgery in Heidelberg, in 1909. They can be driven through bone with a T-handled chuck or a powered drill (Fig. 8.29). They can be introduced at

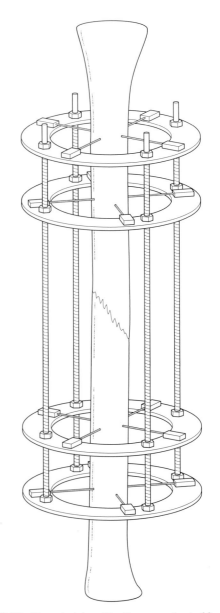

Fig. 8.28 The principles of the Ilizarov method of fixation.

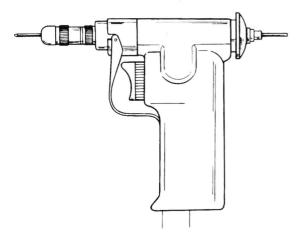

Fig. 8.29   A powered drill to insert wires.

operation or inserted percutaneously. Use a single wire to fix small bones such as phalanges by impaling them as though on a skewer. A number of fragments can be threaded on the wire like a kebab (Fig. 8.30). Use the largest size you can insert without splitting the fragments. Insert several wires in order to prevent rotation of the fragments (Fig. 8.31). Kirschner wires offer a valuable method of stabilizing fragments while you apply permanent fixation.

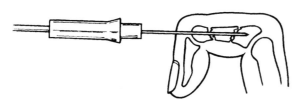

Fig. 8.30   Impaled fragments of a phalanx on a Kirschner wire.

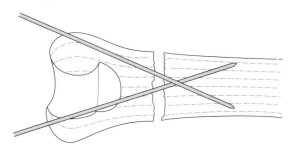

Fig. 8.31   Insert Kirschner wires to prevent rotation of the fragments.

2. Intramedullary fracture fixation has developed from the trifin nail for femoral neck fractures devised in 1931 by the Norwegian American Marius Smith-Peterson and the intramedullary nail for femoral shaft fractures introduced by Gerhard Kuntschner of Kiel in 1940. The principle of the lag screw (Fig. 8.32) produces a stabilizing compression effect. In long bones, locked intramedullary nails can often be inserted with minimal exposure.

BONE GRAFTS

1. Cancellous (L *cancelli* = lattice-work, hence spongy, porous) bone has little strength but has osteogenic potential. A convenient site is the iliac crest. Expose it, detach the external muscles and cut across the crest with an osteotome, leaving it still attached to the internal muscles. Cut thin slices from the exposed edge. Remove the exposed cancellous bone using a gouge, leaving the inner cortex intact. Finally replace the iliac crest and secure it by suturing the muscles over it (Fig. 8.33).

2. Cortical bone is strong and can be fixed in place. However, it is slowly vascularized, may be reabsorbed and has little osteogenic potential. It can be used as a support or strut, to fill a gap.

3. Autografts (G *autos* = self) are usually used since allografts (G *allos* = other) evoke an immune response. This can be reduced by first deep-freezing the allograft at −70°C, but non-union is higher than with autografts. The risk of transmitting viral diseases can be reduced by irradiating the graft – but at the cost of reducing its strength.

AMPUTATION

1. Plan amputation (L *ambi* = around + *putare* + to prune) distal to a joint in order to preserve joint function if possible. This involves retaining the muscle insertions into the distal stump. Preserve sufficient length of stump if you wish to fit a prosthesis on to it.

2. As a rule fashion flaps of healthy skin with underlying tissue, retracted to expose the bone. Single or double flaps are used depending on the vitality and vascularity of the tissues. Divide the fully exposed bone with a saw after protecting all the

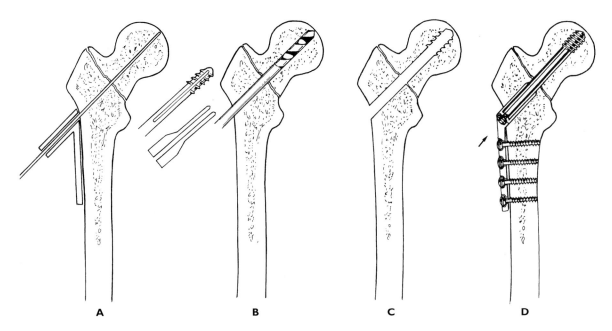

Fig. 8.32   The principle of the lag screw to compress and stabilize a fractured neck of femur. **A** A guide wire is passed and the correct depth is calculated. **B** Next, the track is drilled out. Now the section external to the break is reamed out, while the section internal to the break is tapped (**C**). **D** A lag screw type of pin is screwed into the inner fragment, a plate is fixed to the shaft of the femur and the fracture line will be compressed by tightening a nut threaded on to the end of the lag screw to pull it towards the plate.

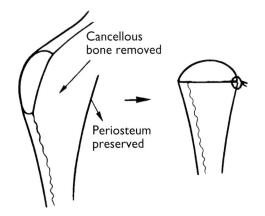

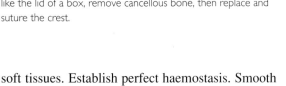

Fig. 8.33   Harvesting cancellous bone. Elevate the iliac crest like the lid of a box, remove cancellous bone, then replace and suture the crest.

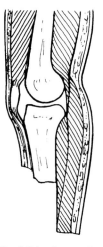

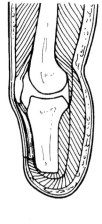

soft tissues. Establish perfect haemostasis. Smooth the bone stump using a rasp.

3. Close the flaps over the stump (Fig. 8.34). Monitor the stump vitality carefully until it is fully healed.

Fig. 8.34   Amputation. This shows a below-knee amputation. Leave the tibia sufficiently long so that a prosthesis can be fitted to it and the knee can be controlled by the descending muscles. The posterior flap has been kept long so that it can be brought over the bone end and stitched to the short anterior flap. Note the rounding of the anterior edge of the tibia.

4. Amputation can often be avoided when a length of long bone must be removed for some tumours. After excising the diseased bone the defect can sometimes be bridged with a graft or metal prosthesis, leaving the limb intact.

JOINTS

1. Certain joints or joint elements can be replaced when they are diseased or damaged.

2. For some fractures of the hip the best treatment may be replacement of the femoral head and neck with a metal prosthesis. The new head and neck are fixed into the femoral medullary cavity by means of a metal stem (Fig. 8.35).

3. Polymethylmethacrylate is often employed to cement the stem in place. As an alternative the stem surface can be coated, for example with sintered metal beads, to encourage direct bonding with the tissues, which grow around the beads, providing a solid fix.

4. For complete hip replacement, the acetabulum (L = vinegar cup) is reamed out to enlarge it and a cup is inserted to receive the replacement femoral head. The head may be of metal, plastic material or

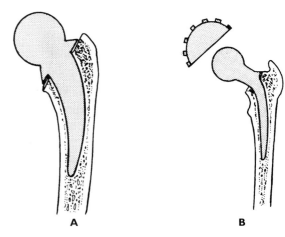

A   **B**

Fig. 8.35 **A** Replacement femoral head which fits into the acetabulum. **B** Total hip replacement. The replacement head fits into a socket fixed into the reamed out acetabulum.

ceramic; this has a low wear rate and its former brittleness has now been overcome.

5. Other joints can be successfully replaced, or the contacting surfaces can be replaced. Small joints, such as those in the fingers, can be replaced using one-piece flexible plastic prostheses.

9

Handling dissection

Organization
Exposure
Sharp dissection
Blunt dissection
Tension
Special techniques
Dissecting round structures
Tissue planes
Dividing tissues
Diseased tissues
Neoplasms
Aids

- Dissection (L *dis* = apart + *secare* = to cut) may be necessary to approach a structure to identify, display, examine, repair or resect it.
- Dissection requires an intimate knowledge of the anatomy and differential make-up of tissues in health and disease.
- Skilful dissection is one of the hallmarks of surgical competence.
- Some surgeons appear to charm the tissues. It is not magic but thoughtful familiarity.

ORGANIZATION

1. Ensure that the patient is in the position that facilitates exposure – supine, prone, straight or flexed.

2. If necessary, have the operating table tilted, provided the patient is properly secured.

3. Make use of gravity. For example, when operating in the pelvis, to empty it of bowel, place the patient head down (the position named after the German surgeon Friedrich Trendelenburg 1844–1925). Alternatively, place the patient head up to ensure that the neck veins are not congested when operating on the neck (often called 'reversed Trendelenburg'). Raise limbs to reduce congestion.

4. Place pillows or sandbags to elevate a part or retain the patient in the required posture.

5. Ensure that you have good, shadowless, glare-free light. In some cases make use of light-carrying retractors and headlight.

EXPOSURE

1. Plan the incision carefully. Do not compromise on attaining safe access but consider the cosmetic and functional effects. Many generations of surgeons have accumulated a wealth of standardized safe approaches. Use a standard approach whenever possible but remember that there are anatomical anomalies and also that disease processes may change the anatomy. In addition, many standard approaches have caveats (L = let him beware, from *cavere* = to take care), such as the need to avoid entering the brachial artery when giving an intravenous injection at the elbow, to avoid injury to the facial nerve when operating on the parotid gland. If you need to use a novel method, study the anatomy carefully, asking yourself why your approach is not normally used.

2. Make sure you are in the correct tissue layer – failure to do so may lead you into error.

3. When possible, gently split muscle and aponeurotic fibres rather than cutting them. You may be able to displace nerves, blood vessels, tendons and ligaments rather than transect them.

4. Make use of the full length of the incision and, if necessary, have the wound edges retracted. Prefer dynamic retraction by an assistant, which can be adjusted as necessary and relaxed at intervals, to fixed, self-retaining retraction. Your assistant can

gently displace intervening structures with fingers, after covering slippery tissues with a gauze swab (Fig. 9.1). Apply tissue forceps to tough structures to retract them (Fig. 9.2)

5. Make use of gravity by moving the patient or a part to displace an obstructing intervening structure. Alternatively use large packs, with tapes attached to substantial metal rings kept outside the wound or clipped to the external towels, to guard against leaving them inside (Fig. 9.3). Sometimes a structure cannot be removed but can be rotated on its anchoring tissues; for example, the left lobe of the liver can be gently folded to give access to the oesophageal hiatus, and the column of trachea, larynx, oesophagus and thyroid gland can be rotated to bring the posterior aspect of the pharynx into view.

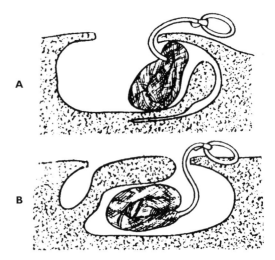

Fig. 9.3   Large packs. **A** The pack holds aside a structure to prevent it from intruding into the wound. **B** A large pack placed behind a structure lifts it up into the mouth of the wound. Note the tapes attached to large metal rings left outside the wound.

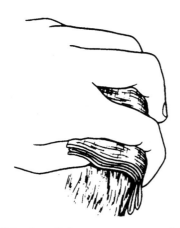

Fig. 9.1   Retracting with fingers over a gauze swab to improve the grip on slippery tissues.

6. Prefer to bring a mobile structure to the surface of the wound in preference to carrying out a delicate procedure in the depths where the lighting and access are limited. Sometimes a pack can be placed beneath a structure to raise it (Fig. 9.3); alternatively, try depressing the edges of the incision (Fig. 9.4).

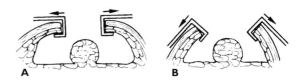

Fig. 9.4   Displaying a fixed deep structure. As an alternative to retracting the wound edges, as in **A**, is it possible to depress them as in **B**?

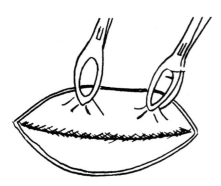

Fig. 9.2   Use tissue forceps to retract tough tissues.

  Key point

- Exposure is prejudiced by poor haemostasis. Blood staining obscures the distinctive appearance of differing tissues. If you wish to see what you are doing, stop the bleeding.

SHARP DISSECTION

1. The scalpel divides tissues with the minimum damage. If the tissues move under the drag of the scalpel, steady them with your fingers, if necessary exerting tension to open up the incision to display the deeper structures (Fig. 9.5).

2. Expertly performed scissors dissection produces minimal damage, especially when floppy tissue is difficult to stabilize for cutting with a scalpel. The blades must remain in contact or they tend to chew through the tissues. Scissors have the advantage that they can be used for blunt or sharp dissection. Insert the closed blades and gently open them to define a plane of cleavage, or cut the tissues to separate them. A potential danger is that in some circumstances the deep blade is hidden (Fig. 9.6), so first carefully inspect and palpate the deep surface.

BLUNT DISSECTION

1. Splitting is a valuable method of dissecting in muscle, aponeuroses and to open up tissues along the direction of linear structures such as vessels, nerves and tendons. It is a method that allows you to follow a natural path rather than create one by sharp dissection. The line of cleavage is parallel to the strong fibres and cuts or tears only weak interconnecting fibres. Scissors can be used to split a sheet after it has been penetrated in one place and separated from deep structures. Insert one blade of almost fully closed scissors into the hole and push them in the direction of the fibres (Fig. 9.7). A different splitting action can be achieved with scissors by holding them perpendicular to the plane of the tissues. Push the closed tips between the fibres and gently open the blades (Fig. 9.8). Alternatively, use artery forceps instead of scissors, since the tips

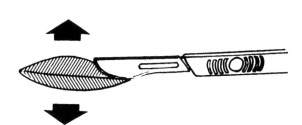

Fig. 9.5 If you apply tension to separate the margins of the incision when cutting with a scalpel, you display the depths of the wound, so you do not inadvertently cut too deeply.

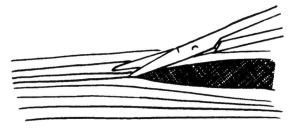

Fig. 9.7 Splitting parallel fibres with scissors. Almost close the scissors and push the small 'V' between the blade tips into the tissues, along the line of the fibres.

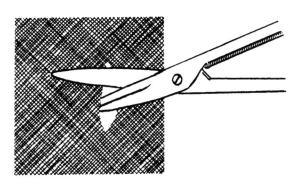

Fig. 9.6 When cutting with scissors, protect the underlying structures from inadvertent damage by the deep blade.

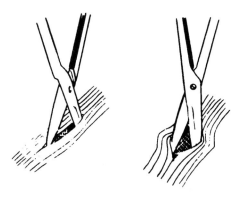

Fig. 9.8 Splitting parallel fibres with scissors. Push the closed tips into the sheet of tissue and open them parallel to the fibres. If there are underlying structures with side branches, open the scissors at right angles to the line of the intended split.

have gently rounded backs. Even more gentle splitting can be achieved by inserting closed dissecting forceps and allowing them to open; the force is limited by the spring of the blades. The handle of a scalpel makes a convenient splitting instrument in some situations.

2. Tearing sounds a crude and traumatic method and so it can be, if employed inappropriately or roughly. Used judiciously it allows you to find the line of weakness, perhaps when two structures are adherent and you do not wish to risk sharp dissection in case you inadvertently cut into one of them. Try inserting two fingers and gently separate them (Fig. 9.9); you have a very accurate feel of the force you are exerting. As you pull the tissues apart, feel and watch carefully to ensure the path of the separation does not deviate.

3. Peeling is valuable when a flexible structure must be detached from another along an adherent tissue plane. Depending on the shape of the attachment, you may use a gauze pledget held in forceps (Fig. 9.10), a finger tip (Fig. 9.11), a finger tip wrapped with a gauze swab (Fig. 9.12) or a swab held in the fingers (Fig. 9.13). Peeling is not wiping, which traumatizes the tissues. If you need to wipe your way through the tissues, you do not know your anatomy.

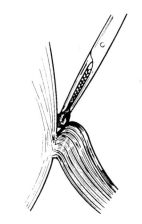

Fig. 9.10   Using a pledget of gauze held in forceps to peel an adhesion.

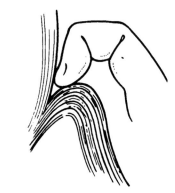

Fig. 9.11   Peeling off a structure using the tip of a finger.

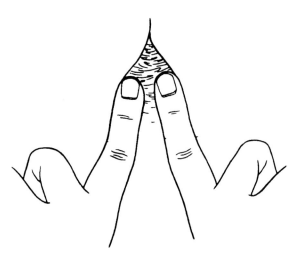

Fig. 9.9   Judicious separation of tissue by a tearing action, trying to sense the correct line of separation.

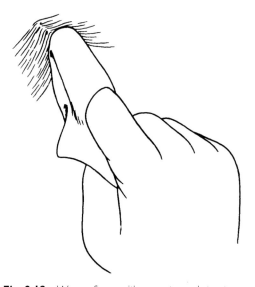

Fig. 9.12   Wrap a finger with gauze to peel structures.

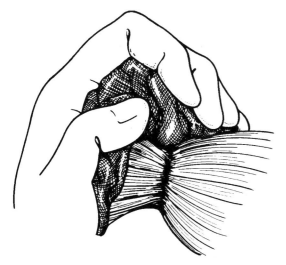

Fig. 9.13 To give you a frictional grip in peeling off a larger structure, hold a gauze swab in your hand.

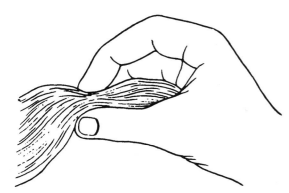

Fig. 9.14 Gently pinch the junction to assess it if you cannot easily visualize it.

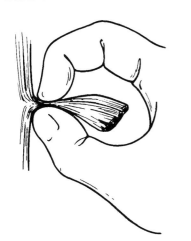

Fig. 9.15 By a combined pinching and peeling action from both sides simultaneously you may be able to separate the tissues safely.

4. Pinching is sometimes valuable when you cannot obtain a view of an attachment in the depths of the wound. You may not be able to view the line of cleavage but by gently pinching the union you can assess the line of fusion (Fig. 9.14) and may be able to pinch it off (Fig. 9.15). The manoeuvre enables you, for example, to detach a benign gastric ulcer that is adherent to, or penetrating, another structure.

TENSION

1. The ability to put tissues under tension is a valuable aid as a preliminary to dissection. It can be exerted by drawing structures apart with tapes, your hands or fingers, dissecting forceps, retractors, packs or tissue forceps (Fig. 9.16).

2. Judicious use of tension aids the identification of attachments and the safest line of separation (Fig. 9.17). By varying the angle of traction you can judge the whole extent of the attachment and test the strength in different areas, since most force is exerted at the edge opposite to the direction of

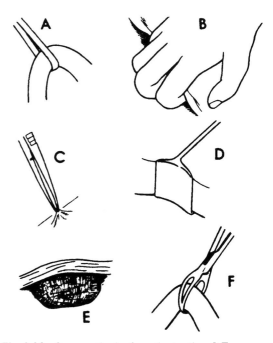

Fig. 9.16 Some methods of exerting traction. **A** Tape.
B Fingers or hand. **C** Dissecting forceps. **D** Retractor. **E** Packs.
F Tissue forceps.

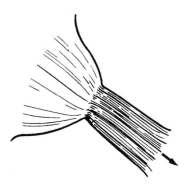

Fig. 9.17 Use gentle traction to test the strength and view the line of attachment.

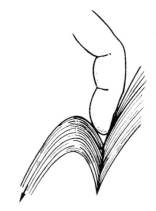

Fig. 9.19 Combined gentle traction and finger-tip peeling will separate the two structures safely.

traction (Fig. 9.18). As soon as an edge begins to separate, change the angle, so that you are constantly working round the attachment, aiming that the last separation takes place at the centre of the union.

3. Be willing to combine techniques. If you apply tension on one structure it may present an edge that you can peel down (Fig. 9.19). A combination of traction and sharp dissection is very effective (Fig. 9.20, 9.21). However, keep changing your line of approach if you encounter difficulty.

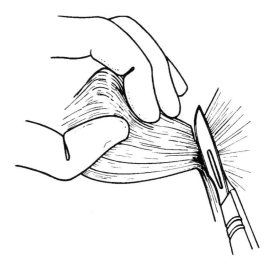

Fig. 9.20 Combined use of tension and sharp dissection with a scalpel is very effective when the attachment is strong.

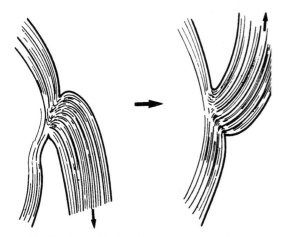

Fig. 9.18 Tension on the attachment is greatest at the point opposite the direction of traction, so you can observe the attachment round the whole circumference and plan the best site for attack.

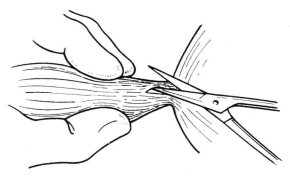

Fig. 9.21 Gentle traction allows you to identify strong bands, which may be isolated and divided with scissors.

SPECIAL TECHNIQUES

1. **Finger fracture** is useful when dissecting in a vascular, friable, solid organ such as the liver. It sounds crude but is very effective. Squeeze a portion between finger and thumb to crush the parenchyma. The larger ducts and blood vessels remain intact and can be doubly ligated and divided.

2. **Ultrasound tissue disruption** is an alternative method to finger fracture. The ultrasound at 20–60 kHz disrupts the cells but the ducts and vessels survive. If the hollow vessels are compressed, they are welded and disrupted.

3. A steady **oscillating diathermy** current applied through a pointed active electrode disrupts the tissues. At the same time, the cut surface is partly coagulated so that small blood vessels are sealed. This is a useful method of dividing large masses of vascular soft tissue such as muscle. Diathermy current can be blended to produce simultaneous cutting and coagulation (see Ch. 10, p. 157).

4. **Laser light** (*light amplification by stimulated emission of radiation*) is an intense, narrow, monochromatic beam. A variety of lasers is available, each having specific characteristics and uses. Laser light may be used to vaporize tissues, at the same time sealing small blood vessels while producing minimal damage to surrounding tissue.

5. **Water jet** disrupts soft parenchymal tissues but the ducts and blood vessels remain intact, to be doubly ligated and divided.

6. **Cryosurgery** (G *kryos* = frost) is carried out by placing a cryoprobe cooled with liquid nitrogen or liquid carbon dioxide against a lesion. The tissues form an ice-ball, which subsequently undergoes necrosis and sloughs off, leaving a clean ulcer. The technique is virtually painless but requires special training.

DISSECTING ROUND STRUCTURES

1. You may need to dissect behind a large structure, either to secure the blood vessels entering and leaving it before excising it, or to carry out a procedure on another structure hidden behind the mass.

2. Ask yourself if you can avoid the problem by using another approach, or reduce the size of the mass – for example, deflate distended bowel or aspirate fluid from a cystic mass.

3. If you encounter difficulty, do not proceed doggedly on. Stop and reassess the problem. Can you approach it from a different aspect, lengthen the incision, improve the retraction, improve the light, further mobilize the intervening structure?

4. Remember that the difficulty is usually greatest at the beginning. As you mobilize the target structure, exposure improves. However, do not forget that the other danger point is at the end, when you may become too casual and spoil a previously painstaking dissection.

5. Choose to start where you get the best view, where you are most confident about the anatomy, where you can best control blood vessels, and where a minor division of the tissues is likely to reap the highest rewards in facilitating further dissection. Of course, not all these aims are fulfilled at a single point, so choose the best compromise.

6. Do not cut blindly. This is almost an inviolable rule. Even so, make sure that you have good control of potential bleeding. Remember, when trying to locate blood vessels, that applying tension is likely to obliterate arterial pulsations and empty veins so that you cannot identify them.

7. When transecting a pedicle underneath an overlying structure, it may be initially easier to transect it as far as possible from the mass, but this may leave the remaining pedicle short and more difficult to secure (Fig. 9.22).

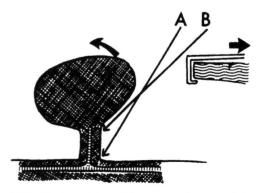

Fig. 9.22 The base of the pedicle is most easily seen at **A**, but the vessels can be better controlled if they are first sought at **B**.

TISSUE PLANES

Key points

- This is, perhaps, the most neglected aspect of dissecting. Intimate knowledge of the correct plane distinguishes the master from the pedestrian surgeon.
- When the anatomy is distorted, once you confidently reach the surface of an identified structure, do not wander from it, because you are then entering an unknown area.

1. For example, when operating on the thyroid gland you need to incise several diaphanous layers delicately, until you see the veins on the gland fill up as the last restraint is removed, confirming that you have entered the correct plane. Similarly, when exposing the vagal nerve trunks at the oesophageal hiatus you need to incise the peritoneum and then the phreno-oesophageal ligament.

2. When you are dissecting near the liver, for example, do not lightly wander from it. It is a valuable marker: its surface is a tissue plane you can follow to reach contiguous structures safely.

3. When opening up an obliterated tissue plane you may know the structure and the strength of the structure on one surface, but do not assume the strength of the tissues that you are separating from it: take great care until you have confirmed its nature.

4. When dissecting along a structure such as a nerve or blood vessel, proceed carefully to avoid damaging any branches, tributaries or other structures. Nerves, arteries, veins and lymphatics often run in parallel.

5. The greatest challenge is to leave the safe plane in order to encompass tissues, such as a malignant tumour, that must be excised together with a surrounding layer of healthy tissue, in such a way that you do not expose or encroach on the tumour, for fear of disseminating the malignant cells. The difficulty is twofold: you must know the normal anatomy and the possible

results of distortion, and you must be able to distinguish normal tissue from potentially malignant tissue.

Key point

- If disease has distorted the anatomy, do not inexorably persist in your intended approach. Try approaching it from different aspects. Also, try starting your dissection from a short distance away in normal tissue and work towards the diseased area.

DIVIDING TISSUES

1. Membranous layers often overlie important structures and it may be impossible to be sure if the underlying structures are attached until you have breached the layer. If the membrane is sufficiently lax, pinch up a fold with your fingers to estimate its thickness and mobility on overlying structures by rolling it between your fingers. Now pick up a fold with dissecting forceps to tent it. Apply a second forceps close by on the tented portion, release and re-apply the first forceps to allow anything caught in its initial grasp of untented membrane to fall away. Have the two forceps held up to create a raised ridge. Make a small scalpel incision on the crest of the ridge to let air enter and allow any structure to fall away (Fig. 9.23). Enlarge the incision so you can insinuate your finger and explore the under-surface of the membrane to ensure that it is clear. Through the entry hole, insert the blades of dissecting forceps, or two separated fingers, under the membrane and cut between them (Fig. 9.24). As you proceed it becomes progressively easier to inspect the deep aspect of the membrane.

2. When it is critically important to avoid cutting more than the membrane, infiltrate the layer with sterile physiological saline to expand the tissues and render them more translucent.

3. If the membrane is the peritoneum and it has been opened previously, always start the new incision just beyond the end of the previous closure, where you can tent it and also reduce the risk of

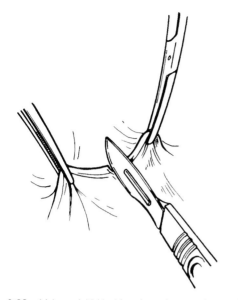

Fig. 9.23 Make an initial incision through a membrane after lifting a ridge with forceps.

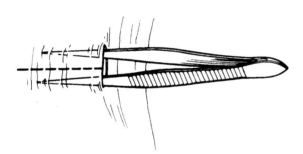

Fig. 9.24 To enlarge a hole through a membranous layer, insert dissecting forceps through the hole and incise the membrane between the blades of the forceps, as indicated in the dotted line.

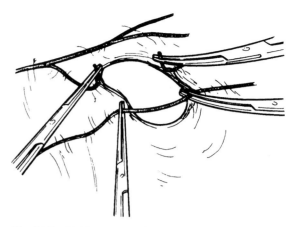

Fig. 9.25 Dividing a sheet of vascular connective tissue. Isolate and doubly clamp the vessels before incising the sheet.

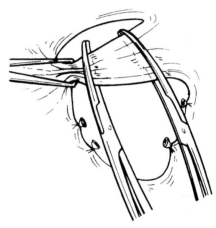

Fig. 9.26 Dividing a vascular membrane between haemostatic clips. The forceps on the right will not grip the full width of the flattened ribbon. On the left the portion of membrane has been bunched with dissecting forceps before clamping it. Note that the left-hand forceps have the tips projecting beyond the clamped membrane, to facilitate the application of a ligature.

cutting an adherent structure. If it is too tense to be tented, infiltrate it with saline to thicken it and allow you to estimate the residual thickness.

4. To divide a sheet of vascular tissue, first doubly clamp major vessels before incising the membrane. The less tissue that is included in the ligatures the less likely they are to be dislodged (Fig. 9.25). If there are few major vessels, you may double clamp, divide and ligate sections (Fig. 9.26). Do not attempt to gather too large clumps within the forceps. Artery

forceps grip well only near the tips. In addition, if vessels lie within bunched-up tissue within a ligature, they can retract and rebleed.

6. If the sheet is very vascular, consider infiltrating it with isotonic saline containing adrenaline (epinephrine) in a concentration of 1:400000 to produce vasoconstriction and reduce oozing. Alternatively, use cutting and coagulating diathermy current.

7. Homogeneous tissue is best divided using clean cuts of the scalpel to produce the minimum

of damage. If possible, apply tension on each side of the incision to open it out and allow you to estimate the depth of the remaining tissue. Make each successive cut along the line of the preceding one in the deepest part of the wound. Tentative, scratch-like cuts create ragged tags. The fibres are sometimes aligned predominantly in one direction. Try to split rather than transect the fibres. If you are likely to encounter an important structure, prefer to dissect parallel to it rather than across it. In some cases you may be able to take the full thickness in successive thin layers so you can identify important structures within each layer. As each successive layer is confirmed to be free from important structures, you can then safely divide it. Create the layers by inserting the closed blades of scissors, artery forceps or dissecting forceps, then open the blades, or allow them to open, to create a space.

7. When seeking a structure within homogeneous tissue, it is often convenient to use a combined technique of cutting and blunt dissection. Remember, if you insert the closed blades of scissors or artery forceps and open them, the force at the tips of the blades is very high.

DISEASED TISSUES

1. Take note of the changes as you approach an area of acute inflammation. Watch out for increased vascularity, oedema, tissue tension and fragility.

2. In chronic disease the fibrous tissue laid down in response to many disease processes is often irregular and opaque, so there is no warning of impending disaster. The connective tissue that normally encloses many important structures may be destroyed by disease. You may suddenly expose the structure and inadvertently damage it.

3. Disease often alters the character of the tissues so that they are not easily recognized. The anatomical features may be distorted, sometimes as a result of contraction of the fibrous tissue that has been laid down, as it matures. This effect is multiplied if the disease is chronic or recurrent, when there is successive deposition and reabsorption of fibrous tissue. Fibrous attachments sometimes draw

out diverticula from hollow organs and ducts, which are in danger during dissection.

4. Remember that the differential strengths of tissues may be changed by disease processes. Tearing, splitting or pinching require you to know which structure will give way. Be very cautious and anticipate incipient tearing in an unexpected area. Structures that are normally swept aside confidently may be adherent, thickened and resistant to blunt dissection, so that you may prefer sharp dissection.

5. Whenever possible, start the dissection in normal tissue away from the worst of the disease and work towards the diseased area, maintaining exposure and identification of important structures throughout.

NEOPLASMS

 Key point

- Do your homework beforehand. Do not hope for the best. The basis of good management of neoplasms is built on the two pillars of anatomy and pathology.

Radical resection of a neoplasm often demands dissection outside the normal planes in order to excise the tumour totally, along with associated channels of likely spread, for example along lymph channels. It is vital to be able to identify warning signs of impending encroachment on the neoplasm or of inadvertently damaging an important structure that should have been preserved.

AIDS

Anatomy
Learn the anatomy of the part. You must know the normal appearance and situation of the structures and the appearance, texture and relative strengths. It is disappointing that many trainee surgeons do not take the opportunity to revise the anatomy before every operation, whether they are performing it or assisting at it.

Palpation

1. If an important structure is likely to be palpable, feel for it before starting. It is valuable to make a habit of feeling the abdomen before starting an operation, when the abdominal wall is relaxed.

2. During the operation feel for arterial pulsations – but remember that tension may obliterate the pulse.

3. Take every opportunity to feel normal and abnormal structures. Until you know the range of what is normal, you cannot confidently identify the abnormal.

Haemostasis

Keep the operative field clear of blood, which obscures the view and stains every structure the same colour. Bleeding is inimical to safe, effective dissection. Prevent potential bleeding, control it when it occurs and remove any blood that collects as a result of bleeding. Do not attempt to work in the depths, in a pool of blood, with continuing uncontrolled bleeding. This is a recipe for disaster. When you are operating on limbs, you may use elevation and a tourniquet to produce a bloodless field (see Ch. 10, p. 157).

Find a safe starting point

In some circumstances you can identify an initial structure that remains your guide.

1. When excising a parotid tumour, first identify the facial nerve emerging from the styloid foramen. You can then follow it as it divides, and preserve it and its branches.

2. Some vessels and nerves have reliable relationships to fixed structures and you can follow them from here. A well-known relationship is that of the long saphenous vein, which can be found reliably 4 cm ($1\frac{1}{2}$") above the tip of the medial malleolus of the tibia.

Needles

If a sought for structure is hard, as for example a stone, try locating it with the point of a sharp needle. Search for a cavity, duct, or vessel containing fluid with a fine-bore hollow needle attached to a syringe to detect if you can aspirate identifiable fluid.

Fluid infiltration

In case of difficulty do not hesitate to infiltrate the tissues with isotonic saline to facilitate the separation of the structures. Fluid renders the tissues translucent, making it easier to see approaching structures. In some circumstances it is valuable to infiltrate the tissues with saline containing adrenaline (epinephrine) in a dilution of 1:200 000 in order to reduce oozing.

Transillumination

Sometimes the structures can be lifted and viewed against a light, or a light can be placed behind them. This allows you to view the vessels – but remember that compressed and emptied veins transilluminate. Always relax the tissues during transillumination. This method is very valuable when you are resecting or joining bowel, since it allows you to identify the supplying vessels in the mesentery.

Probes and catheters

Place a probe in a track or duct that you wish to excise or preserve, as a marker. The technique is valuable during the excision of a thyroglossal fistula. On occasion, it is a valuable help to insert a ureteric catheter before excising an extensive and adherent tumour nearby. You can then often preserve the ureter from inadvertent damage. If you need to resect a portion of it, you can take the appropriate steps to deal with the problem. If you have not marked it, you may be unaware of it and therefore unprepared for the consequences.

Dyes

Some surgeons inject a coloured dye, such as methylene blue, into a complicated fistulous track as a marker. I have not found it very helpful because the dye tends to leak widely and stain all the tissues.

Intraoperative ultrasound scanning

Small probes can be used to help in locating important structures and also to indicate the substance. The combination of ultrasound with Doppler analysis (duplex scanning) allows you to detect blood flow in vessels. The technique has increasing value and is likely to be extensively used.

Flexibility

1. Do not invariably display structures from only one direction. From time to time look from other aspects, especially so if you are in difficulty or uncertain. If you are using tension or distortion of the tissues to facilitate the procedure, relax it from time to time and review the situation with the tissues returned to their normal state.

2. Do not be limited in your technique. Make use of the whole range of possible skills to carry out the procedure safely. For this reason, see as many other surgeons as possible, in different specialities – you may find that you can adapt some of their techniques and instruments to your own practice.

Priorities

Worry about problems in the correct order. Do not become obsessed with one problem at the expense of other considerations. Do not concentrate on details at the expense of important principles. If you encounter difficulty, do not obsessively continue along the path of your original decision; review the possibilities and decide if you should change your priorities. Good surgeons incorporate all their findings into their decisions.

10

Handling bleeding

Definitions
Prevention
Technical aids
Control

- Arteries bleed bright red blood in spurts when cut. They usually constrict and seal if they are transected, provided they are healthy; diseased, calcified arteries cannot contract efficiently.
- Veins ooze dark blood. They can constrict – but do not trust them!
- Capillary bleeding will stop following gentle compression – provided there is no clotting defect.

DEFINITIONS

1. *Primary haemorrhage* (G *haima* = blood + *rhegnynai* = to burst) occurs during operation.

2. *Reactionary bleeding* results in the postoperative period when the blood pressure recovers, or straining raises venous pressure, dislodging respectively arterial and venous clots.

3. *Secondary haemorrhage* is the result of infection, with bacterial dissolution of occluding clots.

  Key points

- Uncontrolled bleeding encourages hasty, illconsidered actions that prejudice surgical success.
- Anticipate and prevent bleeding by correcting anaemia and clotting defects.
- If bleeding is likely, ensure you have ordered adequate volumes of cross-matched blood.

PREVENTION

1. Study the anatomy so you can expose and control major vessels before you cut them.

2. When you encounter an important blood vessel that must be preserved, obtain control by placing across it a non-crushing clamp ready to be closed if necessary, or encircle it with flexible silicone rubber slings or tape (see Ch. 5).

3. If you wish to divide a major vessel, display it, pass two ligatures under it and tie them at a distance from each other, then divide the vessel between them. Alternatively, apply haemostats on each side of the point of division, section the vessel, then ligate each cut end (Fig. 10.1). Do not apply the clamps too close together or the ligatures will be too near the cut ends and may slip off. Sometimes you

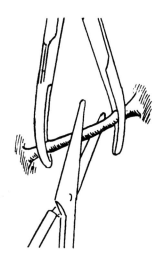

Fig. 10.1 Doubly clamp and divide the vessel. Note that the curved haemostats are placed with their concave surfaces facing each other. This will facilitate the application of the ligatures beneath them.

can achieve sufficient space by applying three clamps, removing the middle one, and cutting through the space left by it (Fig. 10.2).

4. When tying very large arteries, be prepared to place three artery forceps side by side and cut through the vessel leaving two forceps on the proximal stump. Tie a ligature under the deeper of the two forceps and remove it, then tie and tighten a second ligature before removing the second pair of forceps.

5. If an arterial stump continues to pulsate after ligation, it may gradually roll off a ligature. The safest method of avoiding this is to apply a trans-fixion suture–ligature. Pass a needled thread through the artery and tie it to the short end, encircling half the circumference, then take a full turn round the vessel and tie a triple-throw knot. The transfixion prevents the ligature from being displaced.

6. If you are operating on vascular tissues or organs, obtain control of the feeding vessels. You can sometimes apply non-crushing clamps across a soft structure such as kidney or liver, without damaging it, or encircle a portion with a tape that can be pulled sufficiently tight to constrict the vessels without injuring the organ.

7. Be doubly careful when working in the depths, since any bleeding will rapidly create a pool, hiding the site. Take particular care not to injure large veins at sites where they are held open by surrounding structures, as in the pelvis.

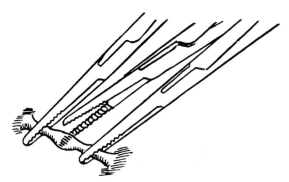

Fig. 10.2 To create sufficient space between the clamps when a short segment only can be exposed, gently apply three clamps side by side and remove the middle one. This ensures that there is a sufficiently long stump presenting beyond the ligatures.

8. Do not open large central veins such as the internal jugular vein unless you have good control. When the patient inspires, air may be sucked into the heart and cause frothing, with immediate circulatory failure.

9. When dissecting in vascular tissues, avoid mass exposure. Prefer to tackle small sections at a time, gaining complete control before proceeding to the next section.

TECHNICAL AIDS

Fluid infiltration

1. This is an effective and often ignored method of reducing bleeding during operations on vascular tissues. Inject sterile physiological saline as you move the needle point, after initially aspirating the syringe to ensure that the needle point is not in a large vessel. The fluid raises the tissue pressure and renders the tissues translucent.

2. In appropriate circumstances, as an extra aid, add adrenaline (epinephrine) 1:200 000 to produce local vasoconstriction.

Tourniquet

1. This is a valuable method when carrying out delicate operations on the limbs.

2. It is contraindicated in the presence of ischaemia, or venous thrombosis from vascular disease or trauma, if the soft tissues are injured or infected, or if there are bony fractures.

3. First empty the limb by elevating it for 2 minutes.

4. Encircle the proximal part with orthopaedic wool and apply a pneumatic tourniquet over this. Secure the tourniquet with a bandage to prevent it from slipping..

5. You may further exsanguinate the limb by applying an Esmarch bandage of thin, flat, elastic rubber, starting at the tips of the digits, overlapping the turns. Run it as a spiral as far as the tourniquet and secure the end (Fig. 10.3).

6. Inflate the tourniquet quickly to 50–70 mmHg above systolic blood pressure for the upper limb and 90–100 mmHg above systolic arterial pressure for the lower limb. Now unwind the Esmarch bandage.

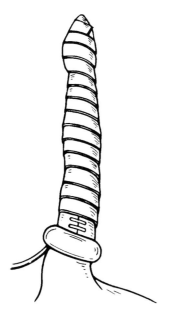

Fig. 10.3 Place a pneumatic cuff proximally round the limb while it is held vertically. Apply an Esmarch bandage from distal to proximal. Inflate the tourniquet and then remove the Esmarch bandage.

7. Record the time of tourniquet inflation and frequently check the pressure. It is conventional to limit continuous inflation to 1 hour for the arm and $1\frac{1}{2}$ hours for the leg. Release the tourniquet for 30 minutes before reinflating it.

8. At the end of the procedure release the tourniquet, so you can ensure that all the blood vessels are sealed, before you close the wound.

Diathermy

1. This is a high-frequency, high-voltage, low-amperage alternating current passed through the tissues. Heating is caused by the vibration of the ions, not by resistance to a high-amperage current.

2. Monopolar diathermy employs two electrodes placed at a distance from each other. Current passes between a large electrode making good contact with the skin and a small active electrode, where the heating effect is concentrated. If contact between the large electrode and the skin is also small, heating will be concentrated here also. Make sure that no earthed metal is in contact with the patient, since this offers an alternative path for the current, especially if there is a break in the normal circuit. Some generators are isolated from earth to increase safety; if the circuit is broken it cannot be completed through earth.

3. It is now recognized that radiofrequency currents induce currents in nearby metal objects even though they are insulated. Any tissue in contact with the metal in which current is induced may be burned. Although this rarely occurs in open surgery, it is well recognized in minimal access procedures.

4. If the alternating current is continuous, tissue disruption at the active electrode has an effect that is similar to cutting, but with some coagulation of the blood vessels. Pulsed alternating current causes desiccation (L *siccus* = dry) of the tissues and coagulation of the blood vessels. The two types can often be blended.

5. Beware of using diathermy soon after applying spirit skin preparation, and in the presence of inflammable anaesthetic or bowel gas, for fear of causing an explosion.

6. Beware of using diathermy current on a patient who has a cardiac pacemaker, for fear of affecting its function.

7. Do not leave the diathermy forceps or needle lying on the patient; keep it in its quiver when not in use.

8. Bipolar diathermy has additional safety because current passes only between the tips of forceps in which the tissue is grasped, and this is coagulated. You cannot pick up tissue in other forceps and merely touch them with the bipolar forceps. Bipolar diathermy cannot be used for cutting.

Laser

1. *L*ight *a*mplification by *s*timulated *e*mission of *r*adiation produces a coherent, high-intensity beam that causes vaporization of the tissues. The wavelength, and thus the tissue absorption, is determined by the medium within which the radiation is generated, such as carbon dioxide, neodymium–yttrium–aluminium–garnet (Nd-YAG) or argon.

2. The heating associated with tissue vaporization produces tissue destruction with coagulation of the small blood vessels.

3. Laser usage demands special training and precautions.

Ultrasound

1. Ultrasonic vibration produces intracellular cavitation, cellular disruption, tissue heating, coagulation and tissue welding, depending on the frequency and power. If a vessel up to 2 mm diameter is gently compressed and low-power ultrasound is applied, it reliably welds and occludes the lumen. At higher power, ultrasound has a disruptive cutting effect and coagulates the vessels.

CONTROL

1. Control generalized oozing with manual pressure, possibly expanded and extended with a gauze pack, or a metal retractor pressing on a pack. Sometimes you can push a pack under a wound edge to exert pressure.

2. Once bleeding has occurred, identify and isolate the vessels, pick them up and ligate them or seal them with diathermy current.

3. If your first clip catches the vessel with its tip alone, it may be difficult to apply a ligature that does not fall off. Do not risk it. Hold the first clip vertically while you apply a second clip beneath it across the vessel with its tip projecting. Then remove the first clip (Fig. 10.4). Make sure, however, that you do not tent the surrounding tissue, lifting a deeper structure into the jaws of the second clip and damaging it. Do not pick up surrounding tissue and ligate it together with the vessel. Your ligature does not directly contact and hold the vessel; arteries can retract, escape from the ligature and continue to bleed.

4. If you inadvertently divide a major vessel, control it initially with direct finger pressure or by compressing the supplying vessel until you have identified it. If you cannot identify the supplying vessel but you know it passes through a particular tissue, try applying a non-crushing clamp – such as a sponge-holding forceps. Do not be hasty: you may wish to repair the vessel. Do not compound the problem by risking injury to other structures. If you can control it with pressure wait 5 minutes timed by the clock. As you cautiously reduce and eventually release the compression you will be surprised and encouraged at how much less dramatic the bleeding is. Do not proceed until you have made sure that you have identified the vessel, assessed the likelihood of further bleeding and confirmed that you have not caused any damage.

5. Prevent calamitous generalized bleeding from happening during a well-conducted operation by proceeding step by step, controlling any bleeding as it occurs. You then have only a single problem on which to concentrate at any time.

6. Tears of vascular organs such as the liver and spleen may sometimes be controlled with sutures but bleeding may continue behind the stitches. Superficial capsular tears are usually amenable to the application of gelatin sponge or microfibrillar collagen powder. Fibrinogen-rich cryoprecipitate can be applied to a bleeding area followed by thrombin, producing rapid clotting.

7. Massive resection is sometimes indicated or, in the case of the spleen, removal of the whole organ; in this case it is important to give the patient

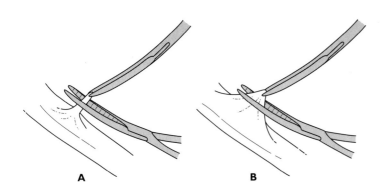

A   B

Fig. 10.4 **A** If you have merely captured the tip of a bleeding vessel with your first haemostatic clip, gently lift it up while you place a second clip across it, with the tip projecting. Now remove the first clip and ligate the vessel. **B** Do not clamp and ligate tissue surrounding the vessel, which could then retract out of the ligature.

polyvalent vaccine, and in the case of children prophylactic penicillin is usually given. These are problems for specialists, since bleeding can often be controlled by interventional radiology.

8. In some cases, simple packing suffices. Use a long pack; start in the depths and lay it back and forth like a jumping-jack firework (Fig. 10.5). After 24–48 hours, return the patient to the operating theatre and, with the same preparations you used for the initial operation, cautiously remove the pack. Again, you may find that the bleeding has stopped.

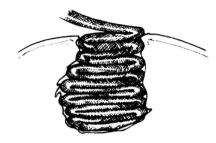

Fig. 10.5 Insert a long pack to control intra-cavity bleeding. Start in the depths and fold it back and forth like a jumping jack cracker. Either close the wound over the pack or bring out the end through the wound. Plan to remove it after 24–48 hours.

 Key point

- When faced with calamitous, life-threatening bleeding, never forget why you are here – to stop the bleeding! Do not get carried away and perform any procedure that is not equally and urgently life-saving.

Intracavity bleeding

1. Unfortunately, you do not have control of bleeding in patients who present having sustained an injury or disease that has resulted in severe, life-threatening bleeding. A typical problem is bleeding within a closed cavity such as the abdomen and chest, since when you enter you may have no idea where the source lies. Tension builds up and eventually reduces the rate of bleeding. When the cavity is opened, tension falls and bleeding starts with renewed force.

 Key point

- When there is bleeding from an unknown source into a closed cavity, defer opening it until you have everything you need to deal with the problem – and have ensured that everything works. As soon as you release the pressure, bleeding will start with renewed vigour.

---

2. Your hand may be forced when bleeding in the chest is causing serious cardiorespiratory distress. Have available a generous supply of large packs, two powerful suckers, large dishes in which to collect the large blood clots and long-handled artery forceps for clamping vessels in the depths. In addition, order vascular surgical instruments and sutures.

3. If you open the cavity and merely suck out the blood you may exsanguinate the patient. Therefore, in the abdomen, open it swiftly and extensively, and insert packs into each quadrant, then pack the central area (Fig. 10.6). If necessary, apply pressure until you have controlled the welling up of blood – but

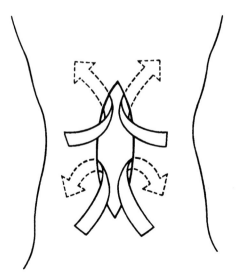

Fig. 10.6 Place large packs into the abdomen to control calamitous bleeding.

remember that compression squeezes out blood from the packs. Do nothing further except to scoop out loose blood and clots that will obscure your subsequent search for the origin of the bleeding, while the anaesthetist resuscitates the patient, restoring the blood volume.

4. If you have controlled bleeding and the patient's condition is improving, adjust your psychological tempo. Do not rush to 'do something'; carefully consider your options and tactics. Be willing to change your mind from your initial intentions. Ensure that you have all the help, equipment and instruments that you are likely to need.

5. Arm your assistant with a sucker from which the guard has been removed. Peel back the edge of the central pack, compressing the part just behind the revealed area. If you see bleeding, isolate the smallest possible area and have your assistant maintain a clear field, using the sucker. Do not automatically clamp a vessel; you may wish to repair it.

6. As you control each area, continue to peel back the pack until you can remove it and start on the pack in the quadrant least likely to be the culprit. When this is finally removed, unpack the next most unlikely quadrant and so on, until, if all goes well, you are left with a final quadrant, having carefully checked and controlled all the others. Try to start at the highest point so that any bleeding will drain elsewhere. You may be pleasantly surprised to find that bleeding has diminished in the interval. Control it while you decide how best to deal with it.

 Key points

- When you have stopped the bleeding DO NOT CLOSE UP! Wait while the anaesthetist restores the blood pressure and improves the patient's general condition.
- Have you removed all the blood that has collected? Stagnant blood makes an ideal culture medium.
- In your efforts to control the bleeding, have you injured or imperilled any other structure?
- Once the bleeding is under control, the situation is no longer urgent.

Handling drains

- The simplest method of removing fluids is to bring the source to the surface as a stoma.
- Drains channel blood, pus, body secretions and introduced fluids, including air.
- Drains uncertainly empty existing fluids.
- When drains have been removed, subsequent collections sometimes emerge from the track.
- Drains unreliably signal the development of complications such as leakage, infection or bleeding.
- Fluids may be brought to the surface from cavities by gravity, suction, *vis a tergo* or capillarity.
- Drains can be used to bring together or keep together surfaces that would be separated by intervening fluids, such as air in the pleural cavity, oozing of blood from apposed raw surfaces.

Key points

- The value of drains is hotly debated:
- Proponents claim they remove harmful fluids, monitor complications, and do little harm.
- Opponents claim they cause irritation, perpetuate discharge and offer an inward track for contamination.

CAUTION

1. In the absence of scientific knowledge or extensive personal experience, use drains where orthodox practice favours them.

2. As a trainee, follow the practice of your chief, but observe the results so you can develop your own views.

3. Use the softest and least irritant materials, ensure the drain does not press on damaged, delicate or vital structures, or suture lines.

4. If possible, bring the drain to the surface through a separate wound rather than the main wound.

5. When possible, make the track lead outwards and downwards to benefit from gravity drainage. If you are using suction drainage, have the drain tip at the lowest point, where fluid is likely to collect.

6. Whenever possible, use a closed system to avoid the possibility of inward contamination.

TYPES OF DRAIN

Packs and wicks

1. Gauze packs are sheets of sterile cotton gauze (Fig. 11.1) placed on a raw surface where discharge is expected to occur over a wide area, such as an abscess cavity or a laid-open superficial fistulous track, or as an initial treatment for an infected

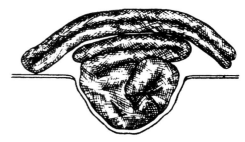

Fig. 11.1 Pack a wound with sterile cotton gauze. Make sure the pack is large enough to absorb the expected discharge. Cover it with dry gauze that should remain dry and not become soaked.

wound. Gauze soaks up fluid most effectively if it is dry but some surgeons prefer it moistened with sterile isotonic saline solution or antiseptic solution.

2. Gauze in contact with raw tissues soon adheres as it is invaded with fibrin threads. You can avoid this by soaking it in sterile liquid paraffin, alone or emulsified with an antiseptic such as flavine. This destroys its ability to soak up fluid, which now tracks between the pack and the raw surface. As an alternative, first lay on a thin non-adherent net of tulle gras (F *tulle* = net + *gras* = fat) or a plastic substitute.

3. The absorbent pack may be overlaid with cotton wool so that it can be compressed by crepe bandage, a corset or elastic adhesive strapping. Compression may reduce oozing and oedema. Since the cotton wool is intended to remain dry and elastic to distribute the pressure evenly, make sure that it does not get soaked or it will form a hard cake; moreover, a completely soaked pack forms a moist channel for microorganisms from the exterior to the raw surface.

4. When the source of discharge cannot be brought to the surface, a wick of folded gauze, or a gauze ribbon, can be passed down to it (Fig. 11.2). It may block rather than hold open the channel. It is fully effective only until the gauze is soaked; thereafter it lies moistly and inertly in the channel. To avoid the wick becoming adherent to the tissues it may be passed through a thin-walled latex tube – a so-called 'cigarette drain' (Fig. 11.3). For very small tracks, twisted threads are sometimes inserted.

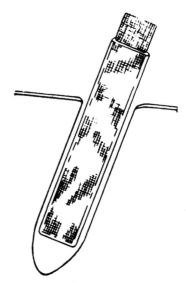

Fig. 11.3 'Cigarette' drain. Pass a folded gauze sheet or ribbon through a thin-walled rubber tube, where it acts as a wick.

Sheet drains

1. A track may be kept open by inserting a sheet of latex rubber or plastic material (Fig. 11.4), which

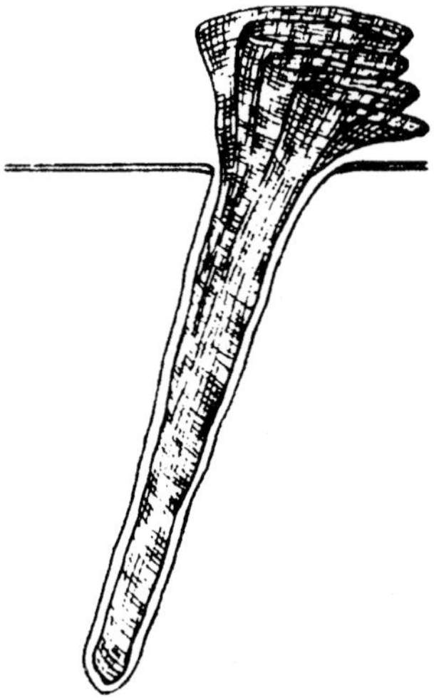

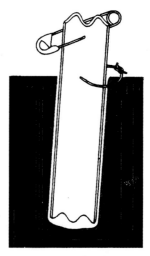

Fig. 11.2 Gauze wick. This is a folded gauze sheet or ribbon, passed down a track to keep the track open.

Fig. 11.4 A corrugated sheet drain of latex rubber or plastic material. It has been sutured in place and transfixed by a safety pin in the projecting portion.

is often corrugated to create spaces. Alternatively, a Yeates drain (Fig. 11.5) is made up of parallel plastic tubes. However, these are inert and fluid reaches the surface by gravity or *vis a tergo* (L = push from behind), where it must be soaked up by gauze packs. Fix them to prevent them from slipping into the wound by stitching them to the skin and also by placing a large safety pin through the projecting portion

2. Although sheet drains are not very effective, they are popular for the drainage of abscess cavities and to provide a track in case there is any subsequent discharge.

Tube drains

1. These have the great advantage that they can lead away any content into a receptacle, such as a bag or other reservoir, thus forming a closed system, reducing the possibility of infection tracking back into the tissues. Tube drains usually have side as well as end holes (Fig. 11.6).

2. When fluid has entered the tube it may stagnate unless the tube is inserted upwards so it can drain by gravity. Fluid will flow only provided it is not viscous and only if the tube is sufficiently wide so that air can displace the fluid. If the tube is too narrow, the force of capillarity tends to retard the flow. However, fluid empties by *vis a tergo* if, for example, it is pushed out by a rise in intra-abdominal

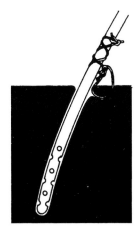

Fig. 11.6 A tube drain with multiple side holes, of silicone rubber or plastic material. Note how it is secured by tying thread back and forth around it, then with a stitch through the skin that is loosely tied. The tube has not been transfixed and therefore will not leak.

pressure. A limb may be compressed with a bandage to express any fluid into a drain.

3. Usually, the most effective method is to apply suction. Insert the tube so the tip lies at the lowest part where fluid is most likely to collect. The tube may be connected to a syringe fitted with a rubber bulb that is compressed before being attached, so that as it expands it exerts suction. A proprietary system uses a bottle that can be evacuated by a vacuum pump, then attached to the tube; the bottle cap incorporates an indicator to signal when the vacuum is lost.

4. The most versatile method is to apply suction directly from an electrically driven vacuum pump, incorporating a reservoir to collect any discharge from the drain. The suction tends to drag tissue into the holes of the drain and block them, rendering the system ineffective. This can be partially overcome by using a pump that automatically and intermittently breaks the vacuum, allowing the pressure to rise to atmospheric – but the tissues may remain trapped in the holes.

The Shirley drain (Fig. 11.7), allows air to leak throughout, drawn in by the suction through a side tube protected by a bacterial filter. However, the most effective method is to use a sump drain (Fig. 11.8). Place a large tube with side holes at the bottom of the

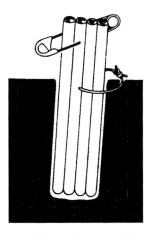

Fig. 11.5 Yeates drain – a sheet formed of parallel tubes of plastic material.

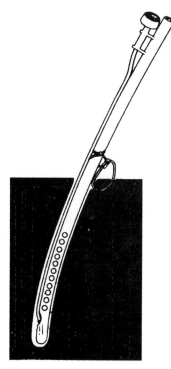

Fig. 11.7 The Shirley wound drain incorporates a side tube guarded by a bacterial filter so that, when you apply suction to the main tube, sterile air can be drawn down to the drain tip, helping to prevent tissues from being sucked into the side holes and blocking them.

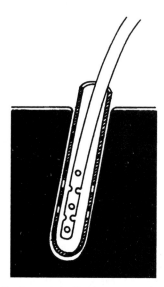

Fig. 11.8 Sump drain. The large outer tube creates a sump in which fluid collects. Lying freely in the bottom of the sump is a smaller tube attached to a sucker. Because the tissues are separated from the holes in the suction tube, they cannot be drawn in to block them.

cavity so that any fluid will collect in it. Lying free within this is a suction tube, which can take up the fluid but cannot be blocked by sucking in tissues.

SITES

Subcutaneous

1. Subcutaneous tissues vary in depth and vascularity in different individuals and in different parts of the body. Blood and reaction fluid collect especially when the skin has been extensively undermined. Small collections can be drained using gauze wicks, corrugated sheet drains or multiple soft tubes with many side holes, connected to a gentle suction pump. These may be preferable to attempting to apply external pressure by means of cotton wool and crepe bandages in the hope of preventing fluid from collecting.

2. In the presence of severe contamination or infection, do not attempt to close the skin, vainly hoping that the drains will provide adequate removal of any discharge.

Subfascial and intramuscular

Do not trust drains in the presence of damaged muscle trapped beneath strong fascial coverings, since fluid collecting here raises the pressure, causing ischaemia, with the risk of infection from anaerobic organisms.

Extraperitoneal

After removing a source of intraperitoneal infection there is a risk of infection of the extraperitoneal tissues. Many surgeons close the peritoneum and leave a drain to its external surface, usually through a separate stab incision. An alternative is to leave the skin wound open and carry out delayed primary closure.

Intraperitoneal

1. This is the subject of bitter controversy. It was shown at the turn of the last century that an intraperitoneal drain is usually sealed off within 6 hours. It is likely that the drain acts as a foreign body and that the discharge consists of reaction fluid in response to its presence.

2. On occasion, intraperitoneal drains continue discharging fluid for prolonged periods if the amount of fluid generated prevents the surfaces from coming together and sealing off. This occurs in ascites.

3. Although drains usually discharge fluid that is already present, the fiercest arguments centre around their ability to channel subsequent fluid collections to the surface and thus to signal a haemorrhage or the breakdown of an anastomosis with subsequent leakage into the peritoneal cavity. It is likely that all the criticisms and claims are correct in some circumstances.

 Key point

> Use intraperitoneal drains, for instance following open cholecystectomy, if it reassures you. Do not, however, allow the insertion of a drain to replace careful performance of the procedure.

---

4. Having inserted a drain do not rely upon it to warn of a leak or a bleed if other features point to a complication.

5. Soft latex drains promote fibrosis and the formation of a track. Silicone elastomer, polyurethane or polyvinyl chloride are inert.

6. Insert drains through a small separate stab wound when possible. Take care to avoid major nerves and blood vessels in the abdominal wall. Keep the track straight by grasping the retracted peritoneum and posterior rectus sheath of the main wound on the side of the drain and draw them towards the opposite side. Now lift the whole abdominal wall upwards, clear of the viscera. Cut straight through the full thickness of the abdominal wall with a scalpel, taking care to cut the peritoneum under vision. Insert straight forceps through the stab wound and grasp the external end of the drain, to draw it out through the stab wound.

7. In some cases it is permissible to bring out the drain at one end of the main wound. If you do so, make sure you use separate stitches to secure the drain from those that close the wound. Eschew this, however, if infected material is likely to be discharged, for fear of contaminating the main wound.

8. Carefully place the inner end of the drain in the most dependent part where fluid is likely to accumulate but make sure there are no sharp ends pressing upon delicate structures.

9. Now insert a stitch through the skin and the drain, and tie it, leaving the ends long. If it is a sheet drain, place a large safety pin through it as an extra safety precaution to prevent if from dropping into the abdomen. If you are using a tube drain, insert the skin stitch, tie it loosely, then take a number of turns round the drain tube, back and forth, tying the ligature on to the drain without puncturing it. The tube drain can be connected in a closed manner, to a collecting bag.

10. Plan to remove intraperitoneal drains after 48 hours unless there is copious discharge. When a drain has been placed very deeply it is sometimes removed by 'shortening it' a little each day.

Pleural cavity

1. Although liquid such as an effusion, pus or blood may be drained, an important function of chest drains is to remove air that has accumulated, has leaked following lung damage or is entering through a breach in the thoracic wall. If the pleural space is occupied by air, the lung is compressed and collapses.

2. Introduce a tube through the chest wall, just above the upper border of a rib, in order to leave undamaged the neurovascular bundle that runs in a groove beneath the ribs (Fig. 11.9).

3. If there is a chest X-ray, examine it to determine the level of the diaphragm on each side, whether the lungs are collapsed and whether there is any liquid in the pleural cavity. From the X-ray and by percussion and auscultation, decide where to insert the drain. You may decide the safest place is the 5th or 6th intercostal space in the anterior axillary line, the 7th or 8th space in the posterior axillary line or the 2nd interspace anteriorly 3–5 cm from the lateral edge of the sternum.

4. You may insert the drain at the conclusion of a thoracic operation under general anaesthetic, or sometimes in the ward with strict aseptic

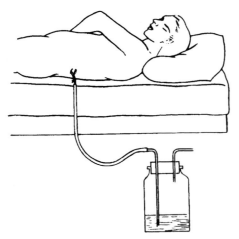

Fig. 11.9 Intrapleural drain with underwater seal. The tubular drain emerges through the chest wall, where it is secured by an encircling but not piercing stitch, which then catches the skin. Connect the tube to the vertical plastic tube passing through the bottle bung, the tip of which lies below the surface of sterile water in the bottom of the bottle. The short, angled tube allows air to escape from the bottle but can be attached to a source of suction.

precautions, after infiltrating the skin and deeper tissues with local anaesthetic.

5. Make a 1–2 cm incision just above and parallel to the chosen rib and gradually deepen it to the pleura. Open the pleura and insert a finger to sweep it round through 360° to ensure that there is no adherent lung.

6. Gently insert a chest drain after removing the trocar; there are side holes, so make sure that they are all well inside the pleural cavity.

7. Insert strong, deep stitches on either side of, but not through, the tube, including the skin. Tie one loosely to seal the hole. Leave the ends long; pass it back and forth around the tube. Tie it after each encirclement, in the fashion of 'English lacing', to grip but not penetrate the tube, preventing it from being pulled out. Leave the other stitch untied and long, to be used to close the wound after withdrawing the tube.

8. Attach the outer end of the tube to sterile tubing that leads to an underwater seal bottle. The tubing is attached to a vertical plastic tube that pierces the bottle stopper and descends almost to the bottom of the bottle, which contains sterile water covering the lower end of the tube. There is another open tube that pierces the stopper and bends at a right angle so that organisms do not fall into it. If necessary, this tube can be connected to a vacuum pump.

9. Place the bottle on the floor.

10. If the intrapleural pressure rises above atmospheric, as the patient exhales, air is forced down the vertical tube and bubbles out through the water. As the patient inhales, a short column of water is temporarily drawn up the vertical tube. During normal breathing the water level in the vertical tube oscillates, signalling that the tubes are patent and functioning correctly.

11. If liquid drains out of the chest it may be trapped in a dependent loop of tubing, damping the oscillation of the level in the vertical tube. Doubly clamp the tube emerging from the chest, disconnect the tubing distal to this, elevate the drain tube to allow the liquid to run into the bottle, then reconnect the tubes and take off the double clamps. Check that oscillation is now normal.

12. You can estimate the amount of liquid draining from the chest by marking the initial water level in the bottle and subsequently comparing the mark with the water level.

13. If air leaks rapidly into the pleural cavity, bubbling will continue in the bottle and the lung cannot re-expand. Check, and if necessary correct, any leakage around the chest drain. If there is none, connect the open tube emerging from the bottle to a vacuum pump set to maintain the pressure in the bottle at slightly below atmospheric pressure. This results in an increase in bubbling but eventually the lung will re-expand, seal against the parietal pleura, and the bubbling will cease. While you are applying suction do not expect to see any oscillation.

14. Intrapleural drains usually seal off and fail to function after 48 hours. You may now cut the stitch attaching the chest drain and withdraw it, tightening, as you do so, the loose stitch to seal off the hole. It is often valuable to apply suction as you gently withdraw the drain so that any last fluid collection is removed. Now tie the loose suture and apply a dressing.

Abscesses and cyst

These are eminently suitable for drainage (see Ch. 12). After you have evacuated the contents the discharge will be small, but continue drainage to allow the cavity to shrink and become partly or completely obliterated. Depending on the site and size of the cavity, you may use open or closed drainage.

External fistulas

1. An external fistula opens on the body surface. Some produce little discharge and do not need to be drained. Others need to be excised or laid open and prevented from bridging over by applying packs.

2. Some fistulas, especially those carrying digestive juices from the gastrointestinal tract, may produce voluminous discharge, which is usually intensely irritant to the skin or excoriating (L *ex* = off + *corium* = skin). The discharge can often be collected in a stoma bag. Cut an accurate hole in the karya gum backing to the stoma bag attachment ring, to fit closely around the discharge site. Clean and dry the skin around the stoma and apply the gum carefully to the skin. The stoma bag ring may have hooks to which you can attach an encircling belt. Clip on the stoma bag. This can be removed as necessary without disturbing the backing ring. In some cases the bag may be emptied from time to time, without removing it, through a tap at the bottom, or by removing and replacing a clip on a spout.

3. Less successful is a box that fits over the stoma, to which suction can be applied to maintain the seal. It works better in theory than in practice.

4. Occasionally, you may be able to pass a Foley-type catheter into the fistulous track, gently inflate the catheter balloon to seal the passage, and allow the catheter to drain into a bag.

Handling infection

The patient
Operation site
Trauma and ischaemia
Bleeding
Viral transmission
Treating infections

In standard textbooks of surgery, infection (L *in* = into + *facere* = to make), signifying invasion of the tissues with living pathogenic organisms, figures at the beginning. I have left it to near the end because all that has gone before has a bearing on infection and the technical factors that encourage it. I shall not deal with sterilization, prophylaxis or antibiotics since these need to be dealt with in depth in comprehensive texts.

The capacity of microorganisms to damage depends upon their virulence and numbers. A relatively small amount of contamination (L *con* = together + *tangere* = to touch), signifying contact with virulent organisms, may overwhelm the defences. Tissues that are healthy, well-oxygenated and uninjured, can survive contamination with many organisms.

Be aware that diabetes, immune suppression or deficiency, alcoholism and many systemic diseases reduce resistance to infection.

THE PATIENT

1. We all have microorganisms constantly with us on our skin, in our noses, mouths and gut. In addition, we may become infected as a result of contact with other people or infected material, especially if we have exposed cuts or injuries or have diminished resistance.

2. Many of the operations we carry out are for the treatment of existing infection. Patients submitting themselves to operation often carry organisms that could be transported to the site of operation. Many organisms are harmless in one site, as in the gut, but are harmful elsewhere.

 Key points

- Eradicate existing infection preoperatively when possible.
- Administer prophylactic antibiotics if contamination is likely or inevitable.
- Administer prophylactic antibiotics if infection is possible in someone who will be at risk because of an pre-existing condition, or someone who has certain implanted prostheses.

3. Hospitals are reservoirs of nosocomial infection (G *nosos* = sickness + *komeien* = to tend, therefore hospital sickness). Moreover, the organisms are often resistant to antibiotics. Many studies have demonstrated that transmission of the majority of infections is by personal contact. This can occur between patients or through nurses and doctors, especially if hand-washing is inadequately performed.

4. Nurses and doctors can become reservoirs of infection to which they may be personally immune. The nose, mouth, respiratory tract, hands and perineum are the most common reservoirs, but instruments, wound dressings, clothing and bedding may harbour organisms.

5. Patients infected with antibiotic-resistant infections are often nursed in isolation – barrier-nursed. Special precautions must be taken by all those visiting them, to limit spread.

OPERATION SITE

1. In the past the skin was assiduously shaved, washed and prepared with sterilizing applications before operation. It is usual now to limit skin preparation to shaving, when necessary, carried out as late as possible before operation.

2. Before making the incision, clean the skin with an antiseptic solution such as 2% iodine in 50% ethanol or 0.5% chlorhexidine in 70% ethanol. Drape the area with sterile towels of linen or proprietary disposable sheets, to isolate the operation site. Some towels cover a wide area and have a central hole through which you make the approach. If you apply several towels, fix them together with towel clips or temporarily stitch them to the skin. Alternatively, or in addition, you may apply a sterile, transparent, adhesive sheet through which you make the incision.

3. You may be operating to deal with an existing infection, or in an area where there are organisms present that are harmless here but would be dangerous if they spread elsewhere. In both cases, take every possible precaution to avoid disseminating the organisms. Pack off tissues outside the immediate area of the operation. Remove immediately or isolate contaminated material. Keep all the instruments used in the contaminated area in a special container, to be discarded as soon as the 'dirty' part of the operation is completed. If it is essential for you to handle contaminated material and tissues to assess them, or as part of the procedure, discard your gloves and replace them with sterile ones before completing the operation.

4. If you encounter infection, always take a specimen or swab for culture and tests of sensitivity to antibiotics.

TRAUMA AND ISCHAEMIA

1. Every surgical operation is traumatic. Do not compound it by handling the tissues roughly. Injured tissues have increased susceptibility to infection as a result of contamination.

2. It is particularly dangerous to introduce, or fail to remove, microorganisms that require little or no oxygen for their metabolism within damaged, dead or ischaemic tissues. Administered antibiotics cannot easily reach them. They may produce toxins that diffuse within the tissues, are absorbed and circulate around the body, often causing specific illnesses.

3. Battle injuries and traffic accidents cause risk of severe infections. Penetrating injuries allow organisms to be carried deeply. High-velocity missiles, especially bullets fired from high-velocity rifles and shrapnel scattered from an explosion, are particularly dangerous. They carry in clothing and other foreign material. If the kinetic energy of the missile is rapidly expended in the tissues, it acts like an explosive, disrupting the cells. Anaerobic organisms will flourish in the resulting dead tissue. For this reason it is essential to remove all dead tissue and foreign material, and expose the retained healthy tissue to the air.

4. Before operation carefully assess the injuries to soft tissue, skin, bones and joints, blood vessels and nerves and the presence of foreign bodies. This allows you to plan your strategy ahead and to order any equipment and back-up that you will need.

5. Under suitable anaesthetic induction, widely open and explore the wound one layer at a time. Gently remove all dead tissue, ensuring that all remaining tissue is clean and viable. Viable muscle should bleed when cut, contract when pinched. Dead muscle appears pale and homogeneous, is friable and does not contract when pinched. Seek and remove all fragments.

6. Make use of lavage with sterile physiological saline to wash out fragments of foreign material.

7. At the end of the operation the whole area should be clean and viable.

8. Should you close the wound?

 Key point

- Do not close a wound if you are not sure if it is recent, healthy, with no foreign material and tension-free.

9. Be willing to lightly pack the wound and wait until it is clean, healthy, free of discharge and then close it, if necessary by applying a skin graft.

10. If you have closed the wound, or if you are dealing with a closed injury, frequently and carefully watch to exclude swelling and tissue tension. This may be most obvious in a limb. If necessary carry out debridement. Incise the skin and deep tissues longitudinally to release the tension. Lay in sterile gauze and replace it at intervals until the wound is suitable for closure or grafting.

11. Mesothelium-lined cavities such as the peritoneal space may be contaminated, as when large bowel is breached surgically, by trauma or disease, releasing organisms within the peritoneum. It may be necessary to create an artificial opening of the colon onto the abdominal wall – a colostomy. Remove every trace of colonic content from the peritoneal cavity with warm, sterile, physiological saline. Once it is freed of contamination the peritoneum is usually well able to resist infection. However, the superficial part of the wound is much more susceptible. You should either drain the superficial layers or leave them open.

BLEEDING

Stagnant blood provides an ideal culture medium for microorganisms. The incidence of wound infection is increased after operations in which excessive bleeding has occurred. Make every effort to leave the operative field completely dry, removing all spilled blood, and guard against continuing or recurring bleeding when the procedure is completed.

VIRAL TRANSMISSION

1. The most important viruses are human immunodeficiency virus (HIV), hepatitis B virus (HBV) and hepatitis C virus (HCV).

2. You can protect yourself and your colleagues by ensuring that you do not risk coming into contact with human blood or blood products and human natural secretions. Make sure you do not sustain, or cause anyone in the team to sustain, skin damage. Be especially careful of needle-stick injuries and injuries with other sharps. Never pass sharps from hand to hand: always place them in a dish whenever they are not being used or when they are being passed from one person to another.

3. Although homosexual males, intravenous drug users and haemophiliacs treated before 1985 are high-risk patients, make your precautions universal. It is dangerous to assume that people who do not fall into the high-risk categories are free of infection.

Operating routines

1. Before 'scrubbing up' check your hands for cuts, abrasions and ulceration. If you find any, apply a waterproof adhesive dressing.

2. During procedures placing you at risk, wear a long apron, an impervious gown, eye shields and double gloves. If your gloves are damaged, change them.

3. Keep all sharp instruments in separate dishes. Never pass them by hand.

4. Avoid spilling blood as far as possible by doubly ligating vessels before you divide them.

5. Use 'no-touch' techniques; operate when possible with instruments rather than fingers.

6. If you sustain a needle-stick injury, encourage bleeding, wash your hands and put on fresh gloves as soon as you can. Afterwards report the incident to the Occupational Health Officer.

7. As a routine, at the end of every operation check your hands for any injuries you may not have noticed while concentrating on the procedure.

 Key point

> 'Universal precautions' means employing safe routines as part of your automatic behaviour. This is particularly true in emergency situations. Do not relax them, thinking 'It will be safe this time'.

TREATING INFECTIONS

Cellulitis, a spreading diffuse infection, usually with *Streptococcus pyogenes*, is not usually amenable to surgical treatment, unless there is a focal infection from which it has spread.

Abscess

An abscess (L *ab* = from + *cedere* = to go) is an enclosed cavity, filled with necrotic material and the products of liquefaction, consisting mainly of dead phagocytes, to form pus (G *pyon* = L *pus*).

1. If it forms near a surface it may eventually 'point,' spontaneously rupture and discharge the pus to the surface of the body, to an internal space such as the peritoneal cavity or into a hollow viscus such as the bowel. At first the swelling becomes reddened, hot and tender. The centre turns first white as the tension compresses and empties the blood vessels, then darkens as it undergoes necrosis. You can usually detect a point of maximal tenderness and softening over a small superficial abscess, and elicit fluctuation in a larger cavity.

2. Local anaesthesia is less effective in the presence of inflammation but in many localized situations it spares the patient the need of a general anaesthetic. If you intend to employ it, raise an intracutaneous bleb in adjacent uninflamed skin and slowly and gently inject ahead of the needle until you have reached the pinnacle of the abscess. If you are impatient and inject under pressure, raising the tissue tension, you will cause pain. If you do not wait long enough for the anaesthetic to take effect, you have wasted your time and will hurt the patient. Never incorporate adrenaline (epinephrine) with the local anaesthetic or you may cause extensive necrosis.

In the case of a finger pulp infection, if you create a ring block at the base of the finger you must avoid at all costs creating a constricting ring of swelling or the whole finger may undergo necrosis. Inject only within the web space, where the volume of fluid will not have any constricting effect.

3. Incise an abscess at the point of greatest tenderness, or on the pinnacle of the swelling. Obtain a specimen as well as a swab for culture and determination of antibiotic sensitivity. Clean out the contents, taking a specimen for culture. If you have any doubts about the aetiology excise a portion of the edge for histological examination.

4. Empty the contents not by squeezing, which will introduce organisms into the blood stream, but with a scoop, or by washing out with fluid from a syringe. Squeezing of infected lesions is particularly deprecated on the face around the nose and upper lip. Organisms will drain by the anterior facial vein into the cavernous venous sinus and may cause thrombosis.

5. Unless this is an obviously small local abscess, insert a finger or an instrument to explore the interior for loculations (L *loculus* = diminutive of *locus* = place) or track. Collar-stud abscess is notorious in the neck when a diseased lymph node undergoes necrosis and liquefaction; the resulting pus then tracks through a hole in the deep fascia to form a subcutaneous abscess. Tuberculous cervical lymph node is a well-known cause. An infected branchial cyst may also create a collar-stud abscess.

6. An abscess near the anus may develop from an infected anal gland, presenting close to the anal margin. An ischiorectal abscess, developing higher up, usually presents laterally and further away. You may be able to feel and open up loculi and detect an upward extension with a finger in the abscess cavity. Do not attempt to probe it in search of an internal opening.

7. An intra-abdominal abscess usually results from localized disease that has been limited from spreading by adhesion of surrounding structures. A typical condition is appendix abscess. When the appendix becomes inflamed, surrounding structures may become adherent and form an appendix mass. If the appendix then ruptures, it does so into a constrained cavity. You need to be very cautious and gentle in approaching the mass for fear of releasing the contents into the general peritoneal cavity, or of damaging any of the viscera forming part of the wall of the mass. Be content to drain the abscess unless the appendix is easily found within the cavity and can be removed without disturbing the other structures.

8. Some other abscesses within the abdomen, which have an underlying cause, may not settle after you drain them. Leakage from a viscus may continue and a track will form to the surface, creating a fistula (see Ch. 4, p. 79).

9. Having emptied the abscess you need to maintain drainage. A wick or ribbon of gauze is sometimes inserted into a small abscess. Very often, this merely acts as a plug. The drain should keep the wound open until the cavity is completely empty, and in some cases until it has had time to shrink and fill up with granulation tissue. Therefore, prefer soft latex corrugated sheet, usually held by a single stitch. If the cavity is deep, insert a safety pin into

the projecting portion as an extra precaution so that it cannot fall into the cavity.

10. If possible arrange that the drainage hole will be dependant so that the cavity will drain by gravity. This may be difficult in the breast. It is rarely necessary to make a second incision from the under-surface of the breast to drain a high, deeply placed abscess.

Boil

A boil (OE *byl* = an inflamed swelling) is an infection of a hair follicle, usually by *Staphylococcus aureus*, and may develop into a small abscess. It does not usually require surgical treatment. Very occasionally it is necessary to incise one that is large and painful without discharging spontaneously.

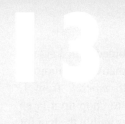

Handling minimal access surgery

with Adam Magos

- Minimal access procedures are feasible because of advances in diagnostic imaging that make extensive exploration less necessary.
- Technical development of lighting, miniature cameras and instruments has extended the range of procedures amenable to minimal access surgery.
- Some operations, notably cholecystectomy, some thoracoscopic and arthroscopic procedures, are generally accepted to be preferable on balance because of reduced hospital stay and earlier return to normal activity.
- The reduction in pain following minimal access procedures, compared with conventional open access, is well established.

1. The German physician Kalk was the first to use multiple access points to obtain liver biopsies but his countryman, the gynaecologist Kurt Semm of Kiel, is considered the father of the technique.

2. Wherever a cavity exists or can be developed, it may be expanded to create a space within which the contents can be inspected, and a wide, and rapidly increasing, variety of surgical procedures can be performed

3. Space in a pre-existing cavity is usually created with the gas carbon dioxide, introduced through a valved cannula from an insufflator that delivers it at a predetermined rate to the required volume, up to a preset pressure, sounding an alarm if this is exceeded. For arthroscopy, distension is achieved with saline. For some procedures, a space can be developed by inserting and inflating a balloon.

4. The main cannula allows the introduction of a combined light source and telescope, attached to a miniature camera and television monitor showing a magnified view. Through separate valved cannulae, various instruments can be freely introduced and withdrawn. Because they are manoeuvred across rather than along the line of sight, their spatial relationships with the target structure can be accurately judged.

5. A disadvantage of the technique is that, as a rule, the target structures can be seen from only one aspect. Since you are not viewing the procedure directly it is necessary for you to learn to coordinate what you see on the screen with your hand movements.

6. The instruments are long-handled and slide in and out through the fixed entry portal, which forms a fulcrum. As the instruments are withdrawn and advanced, the relationship is changed between the inner and outer portions, so changing the amount of movement produced at the tip of the instrument resulting from a standard movement of the handle (Fig. 13.1). The tip can be moved anywhere within a cone whose apex is at the body wall. The shaft of modern instruments can be rotated and fixed in any orientation to the handles so you can hold your hands in the most natural position whatever the direction in which the tip is pointing. However, the functional part of grasping forceps or scissors can be temporarily directed by supinating and pronating your hands.

7. You may be performing an action with an instrument held in one hand while holding the tissue using an instrument controlled by the other hand, or both hands may be simultaneously carrying out complementary actions. Because your hands are often widely separated, they cannot be held as steady as they would be during open surgery, when

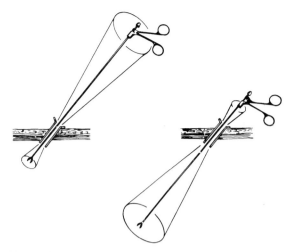

Fig. 13.1   The effect of withdrawing and advancing an instrument through the access port on the volume of accessible space and also the relative effects of movement of the handle on movement of the instrument tip.

the base can usually be brought close to the point of action (Fig. 13.2).

8. Graspers, forceps, scissors, retractors, suckers, irrigators, diathermy hooks and forceps clip applicators, staple applicators and other newly developed instruments are available. Many of them can rotate along the long axis in relation to the handle. It is time-consuming to change instruments and for this reason some of them are designed to be multipurpose, for example combined diathermy hook, irrigator and sucker.

9. Because multiple access ports are used, you can delegate to assistants responsibility for some instruments. The most experienced assistant takes charge of the camera. Some surgeons use voice-directed, body-movement- or eye-movement-directed control in the absence of an experienced assistant. Retraction and steadying of tissues can be delegated to another, and a number of versatile retractors and graspers have been designed.

10. Excised tissues can sometimes be withdrawn through the largest port site, or through a surgically enlarged port site or fresh incision. In women you can create a posterior vaginal colpotomy. A useful method is to place the tissue within a strong, flexible bag, bring out the neck of the bag through a small

exit hole and exert traction combined with a side to side motion to draw it out. Alternatively, a morcellator (F *morceau*, cognate with *morsel*, from L *mordere* = to bite) can be used to chop up a large piece of tissue into small particles within the bag for withdrawal through a small exit port.

REQUIRED SKILLS

1. You need new skills for minimal access procedures beyond those you have acquired for open surgery. Some surgeons find it difficult to adapt.

2. Instead of looking directly at the target area, you watch on a flat screen. On the screen you can see the tips of the instruments in relation to the tissues from one aspect only.

3. You need to learn how the movements of your hands transfer to the tips of the instruments and practise until your movements are instinctive.

4. Since the instruments hinge on the fulcrum of the entry ports, in order to move the tip in one direction you need to swing the handle in the opposite direction.

5. The amount of movement at the tip varies with hand movements depending on the relative lengths of the shaft inside and outside the ports.

6. In open surgery your hands are close to the point of action of the instruments and are able to feel and assess the tissues. Now they are at the ends of long shafts well away from the 'business' ends. Instead of your hands being close together, working in harmony, they are often wide apart at the ends of outstretched arms. Co-ordination of hand movements is difficult to achieve in this unnatural posture.

ACQUIRING SKILLS

1. Courses on laparoscopic surgery are excellent but you cannot acquire skills simply and solely by attending them. They can show you only what to do. You must then go away and practise assiduously until you can perform the movements automatically.

2. Every laparoscopic unit should have simulators where trainees can spend spare time acquiring facility with the techniques.

3. Take every opportunity to handle the instruments and learn the techniques.

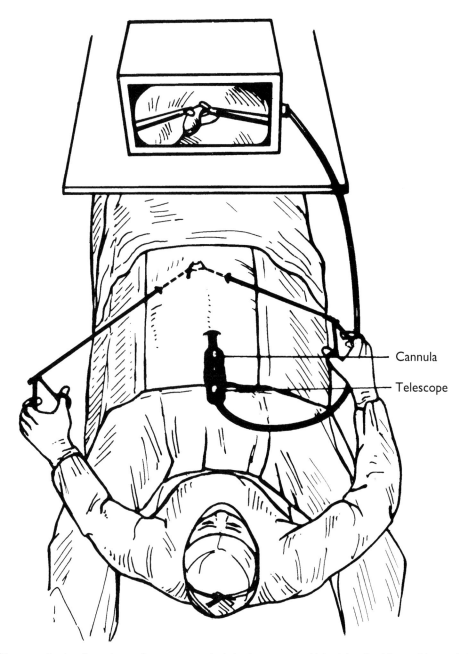

Fig. 13.2 Diagrammatic view from above of a surgeon manipulating instruments with both hands while watching a television monitor showing the view on the camera connected to it.

 Key point

- Skill is not merely knowing what to do, it is being able to do it competently, automatically.

4. You can provide yourself with a simple simulator, using cleaned, worn-out or disposable instruments (Fig. 13.3). Start by placing objects in an open-topped box with direct viewing. Practise picking up objects from one container and placing them in another, using first one hand and then the

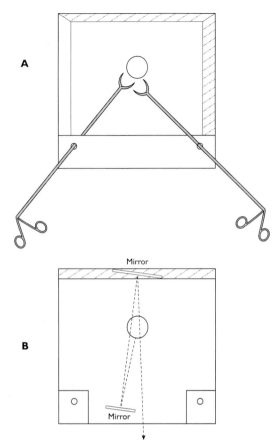

Fig. 13.3. Simple 'home-made' boxes with which to practise minimal access surgery. **A** Remove part of the lid so that you can view the target and instrument tips directly. **B** Place two mirrors so you view the target area indirectly. Place a screen so that you cannot see the target directly.

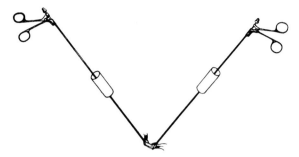

Fig. 13.4 Hold a structure steady using forceps held in one hand while cutting it using scissors held in the other hand.

other. Next, practise picking up objects, transferring them to forceps held in the other hand, then into the second container. Vary the placing of the containers so you need to alter the length of forceps introduced into the box, thus altering the site of the fulcrum and the relationship between hand movement and instrument tip movement.

5. Practise each procedure viewing directly and, when you have become adept, repeat it viewing it with a camera and monitor screen. If you do not have access to a camera and monitor, simulate indirect viewing of the interior of the box using two mirrors.

6. Practise holding a structure with forceps held in one hand after manipulating it to present it most advantageously, and cutting it with scissors held in the other hand (Fig. 13.4).

7. Practise dissection using, for example, a chicken leg.

8. Practise ligation, using multifilament threads which do not have memory. Carry the thread around the simulated cut blood vessel stump. Knotted loops are available commercially, or you can create a Roeder knot (Fig. 13.5). Place the loop over the end of the stump representing a cut blood vessel and tighten the knot by pushing it down the standing part of the thread with a pusher.

9. Also practise doubly ligating and dividing a thread bridging across a space to represent an intact vessel. For this you must tie a standard reef knot. You can form each half-hitch outside the cavity and pass one end through a pusher to tighten it (Fig. 13.6) – in practice your assistant will place a finger over the end of the port cannula to reduce leakage of gas from the abdomen. For this technique you need to pass one end of the loop through the access port, around the structure to be ligated, then draw the end out, where you form the half hitch.

10. The most versatile knot is formed within the cavity in the same way that you form an instrument-tied knot during open surgery (see Ch. 3, pp. 27–29). Remember that grasping threads with metal instruments severely weakens them, so hold them in parts that will be discarded.

11. Practise suturing using a laparoscopic needle holder controlled with one hand and forceps

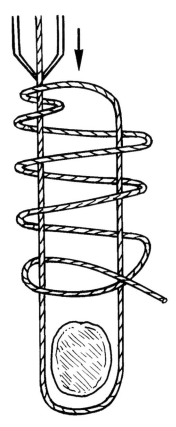

Fig. 13.5 The Roeder knot for tightening a loop. The standing part has been led to the exterior within a hollow pusher rod sitting in the port cannula. Place the loop over the structure to be ligated and tighten the ligature by pushing the knot down using the pusher rod, against counter tension on the standing part. When it is tightened the knot will not slip. Cut off the standing part and withdraw it with the pusher rod.

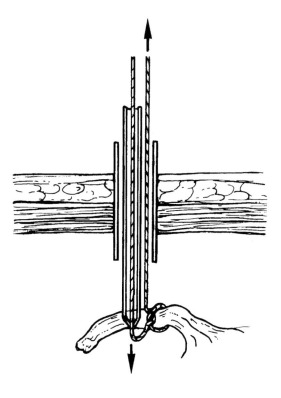

Fig. 13.6 Form a half-hitch outside the abdomen, pass one end through a hollow pusher and tighten it by pushing the hitch down with the pusher against counter-tension exerted on the other thread. Repeat this for subsequent half hitches.

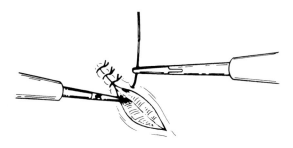

Fig. 13.7 Sewing within a cavity. The needle may be straight, curved or straight with a curved tip – the 'ski' needle.

controlled with the other hand, taking the place of dissecting forceps used in open surgery (Fig. 13.7). Needles may be curved, straight or straight-shanked but with a curved tip, like a ski. Because the needle holder has a fixed point of entry, it must be carefully placed. As you insert the needle, use the other forceps to give counterpressure, to steady the emerging needle without damaging the tip, since you may need to adjust the position of the needle holder on the needle. After drawing through the needle and spare thread, you must encircle the needle-holder with a loop of standing thread, through which you pick up the end of the thread, in order to form and tighten each half-hitch.

 Key point

- Do not forget the principles of correctly forming and tightening knots so they lie correctly, that you acquired in open surgery.

LAPAROSCOPY

1. Laparoscopy (G *lapara* = flank or loins, from *laparos* = soft, loose, + *skopeein* = to view) is normally carried out under general anaesthesia.

2. Obtain consent for the procedure to be converted to an open operation if necessary.

3. Make sure the bladder is empty; if necessary, pass a catheter.

4. If the stomach is distended, pass a nasogastric tube.

5. Carefully palpate the relaxed abdomen to identify any masses and locate the sacral promontory. Percuss the abdomen to detect the lower level of liver dullness.

6. Two methods are available for inducing pneumoperitoneum. The closed method was popular but is being overtaken by the open method on the grounds of safety.

Open pneumoperitoneum

1. Make a 1.5–2 cm incision, either vertical just below the umbilicus or transversely subumbilical. Carry it down to the linea alba, identified by the white fibres after which it is named (L *albus* = white). Other sites may be more appropriate if there are nearby scars on the abdomen.

2. Incise the linea alba, leaving the peritoneum intact to be tented and incised separately, or grasp and lift the linea alba on each side with strong forceps while you cut through it and proceed to open the peritoneum.

3. Insert a finger and sweep it in a full circle to confirm that you have reached the peritoneal cavity and that there are no adherent viscera.

4. Grasp the edges of the incision and insert two strong, 0 monofilament polyamide or polypropylene stitches, taking a good bite of the linea alba and peritoneum, one above the centre of the incision, one below the centre. Capture the untied ends in forceps. Alternatively, insert a single stitch as a purse-string, encircling the centre of the incision and capture the untied ends.

5. Insert a 10 mm diameter cannula. This may be a Hassan cannula, which has a blunt obturator and a conically shaped neck intended to effectively block the entrance hole to stop leakage, a standard cannula with a blunt obturator or a standard cannula with the trocar removed. Some cannulas have an encircling inflatable balloon to fit just beneath the peritoneum, to prevent leakage of gas from the abdomen.

6. Draw the stitch or stitches tight, tie them around the cannula and loop them over the gas inlet. Do not knot the threads but clip them, so you can use them to close the incision at the end of the procedure.

7. Gently ensure that the cannula moves freely.

8. If all is well, connect the gas inlet to the insufflator (L *in* + *sufflare* = to blow), which is set to deliver carbon dioxide at 1 litre/min and against a pressure not exceeding 12–15 mmHg.

9. Switch on the insufflator and check the pressure. If the needle tip is in the large peritoneal cavity the pressure should be not exceed 8 mmHg, with gas flow at 1 litre/min. If you have entered a closed space the pressure will rise above this. Percuss over the liver to confirm that liver dullness has been lost. If all is well, continue insufflation until 3–5 litres have been introduced, provided the abdomen is evenly distended.

10. Pass the telescope, view the interior and check that there has been no damage.

11. Now insert the secondary ports under vision. Swing the combined cannula and telescope so the light lies just under the abdominal wall at each site. View the transilluminated wall to identify any large blood vessels so you can avoid puncturing them. If you need to insert lower abdominal ports, view the inferior epigastric vessels from within, in order to avoid damaging them.

12. Hand over control of the camera to your assistant with instructions to keep in view the entry through the peritoneum of each trocar and cannula.

13. Depending on the procedure to be carried out, place the entry sites carefully. The sites are standardized for most commonly performed operations but they may need to be modified to take into account the shape and size of the abdomen and the presence or absence of previous scars.

> ## 🔑 Key points
>
> - If the entry port is too close to the target structure, the distance between the fulcrum at the port entry through the abdominal wall and the point of action is small, and the cone within which the tip can be moved is restricted. Moreover, a large movement of the handle has to be made to produce a small movement of the instrument tip.
> - Conversely, if the entry port is too far away from the target structure, a small movement of the handle is magnified at the tip, prejudicing fine manipulation.

14. As a rule you will have one monitor, with a second monitor visible to the nurse and to the assistant controlling the camera.

15. You may have a second assistant who has the task of helping the display by retracting and displacing the tissues.

Closed pneumoperitoneum

1. Check the Veress needle (Fig. 13.8). Ensure that the spring-loaded hollow, round-ended, internal cannula will protrude as soon as the outer sharp needle pierces the peritoneum. The side hole in the cannula through which gas can be released into the abdominal cavity must be visible within the bevel of the needle.

2. Make a small vertical sub-umbilical incision for preference, or a transverse incision just below the umbilical scar, and carefully carry it down to, but not through, the peritoneum. Pick up the abdominal wall and gently insert the Veress needle through your incision, into the peritoneal cavity. Feel and listen for the slight click as the internal cannula is released, signifying that you have entered the peritoneal cavity.

3. There are a number of ways to check that you have safely entered the peritoneal cavity, particularly useful if the abdomen has been previously opened. Open the tap of the Veress needle and place a drop of sterile saline on the open Luer connection; the drop

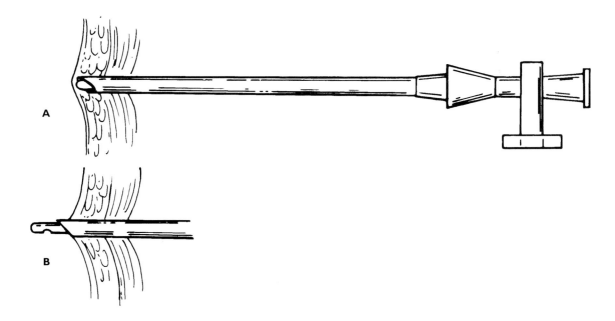

Fig. 13.8 The Veress needle. **A** The needle is just about to pierce the inner lining of the cavity. **B** As soon as the needle has entered the cavity the round-ended, spring-loaded obturator projects, pushing away any structure that might be punctured by the sharp needle and exposing the gas inlet.

should be drawn into the needle when the patient inspires. Attach a syringe containing 10 ml of normal saline and gently inject it, then attempt to aspirate it; if you can recover it, the needle tip must be in a closed space, not in the cavity of the peritoneum.

4. If all is well, connect the insufflator to the needle and cautiously inflate the abdomen.

5. Now withdraw the Veress needle and enlarge the incision down to the peritoneum to accept the trocar with its cannula. As a safety precaution, as the trocar tip pierces the peritoneum, a spring-loaded collar projects, extending beyond the sharp tip on disposable trocars. The cannula has a flap or trumpet valve to prevent gas from leaking. Connect the cannula to the insufflator. Hold the cannula with the palm of your hand, maintaining the trocar in place and with your index finger extended to limit the extent of the initial penetration (Fig. 13.9). Insert it

with a twisting motion, listening and feeling for the slight click as the collar on the trocar extends. You should direct the tip of the trocar downwards, below the previously identified sacral promontory, pointing towards the anus. Distension of the lower abdomen can be increased as you insert the trocar and cannula by exerting pressure in the epigastrium.

6. Withdraw the trocar and replace it with the combined light carrier, telescope and camera attached to the light source and television monitor.

7. Check the abdomen in an orderly and assiduous manner to exclude any damage to the abdominal contents.

Diathermy

1. There are special dangers associated with the use of diathermy current in minimal access surgery.

2. Because the field of view is restricted, you may not notice that tissue outside the intended area of use has been burned by inadvertent contact with the diathermy hook, or via metal in contact with the diathermy applicator.

3. When two metal instruments or structures are in close proximity and the alternating diathermy current is passed through one, it may induce a current in the other, even though they are insulated from each other, and so the current may reach the patient via this route.

> **Key point**
>
> Use the lowest effective power setting. Prefer bipolar to monopolar diathermy if it is available. Select the cutting, rather than coagulation setting.

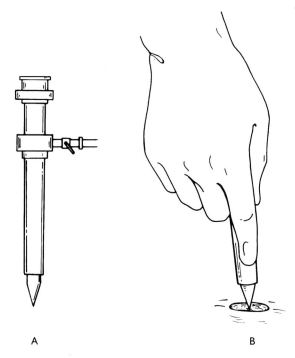

A   B

Fig. 13.9   A The cannula has the sharp trocar in place. **B** The head of the trocar sits in the palm of your hand and your index finger extends along the shaft of the cannula to prevent too deep penetration. Aim the trocar towards the anus, i.e. below the previously identified sacral promontory, using a gentle twisting motion.

Closure

1. At the end of the procedure, first carefully check that there has been no inadvertent damage, no residual bleeding, and no free bodies left in the peritoneal cavity.

2. Remove each instrument in turn while observing the withdrawal from within, to guard against herniation into the defects.

3. Close each secondary port hole after ensuring

that there is no bleeding within the track. Inject bupivacaine into the surrounding tissues and close the fascia using interrupted stitches. Insert a single subcuticular synthetic absorbable stitch, then close the skin with adhesive strips.

4. Finally withdraw the laparoscope under vision

5. Gently compress the abdomen to expel any residual gas.

6. Elevate the margins of the telescope portal by means of the stitches inserted at the beginning of the procedure, and tie them after ensuring that no abdominal contents have insinuated themselves into the gap. Close the skin with adhesive tape.

Other procedures

1. Because of the pioneering work of Kurt Semm of Kiel in Germany, gynaecologists utilized minimal access techniques before general and other surgeons and have extended the number of procedures that can be carried out by the technique.

2. Urologists pioneered many single channel techniques because of the early development of the cystoscope and have adopted minimal access procedures.

3. Orthopaedic surgeons face the problem that joint spaces are difficult to develop. Instead of using carbon dioxide they use saline. As a rule arthroscopy is carried out using general anaesthesia because it is usually necessary to manipulate and distract the joint.

4. Thoracoscopic access allows a number of procedures to be performed, including sympathectomy.

5. Neurosurgeons have also embraced minimal access techniques in many areas.

Index

Note: Page references in *italics* refer to Figures; those in **bold** refer to Tables

gelatin sponge   158
Gillies's combined needle-holders   *10*
glands   127
glycomer 631 thread   17
Gosset self-retaining retractors   *12*
gouge   131, *131*
grafts   109–12, *110–11*
    bones   140
    full-thickness   111–12
    split-skin   109–11, *110–11*
granny knot   19, *19*
grasping forceps, flexible   *64*
guide wires   54–5

haemorrhage
    primary   155
    secondary   155
haemorrhoid injection   60
haemostasis   153
haemostatic clips   12–13
haemostatic forceps   8–9
haemostats   8–9
half-hitch   19, *19*
hands   2
heart   127
hepatitis B virus (HBV)   171
hepatitis C virus (HCV)   171
hip replacement   141, *141*
hook retractors   *12*
hooked wire marker   118
human immunodeficiency virus (HIV)   171
hypovolaemia   81
hysteroscope   60

implantation cyst   79
incision   103–4, *103–4*
incision biopsy   117–18
infantile hypertrophic pyloric stenosis   76–7
infection
    bleeding   171
    ischaemia   170–1
    operation site   170
    patient   169
    trauma   170–1
    treatment   171–3
    viral   171
inflammation, skin   101
inkwell effect   75
interrupted stitches   39, 40
intubation   44–52

direct   48–51
percutaneous   44–8
tracheal   49–50, *49*
urethral catheterization   50–1, *51*
see also catheters
ischaemia   170–1
ischiorectal abscess   172

Jamishidi needle   130
joints   141, *141*

kidney   126
Kirschner wire   139, *139*
knot pull strength test   34
knots   18–34, 88–9
    granny   19, *19*
    half-hitch   19, *19*
    laying and tightening   29–34, *29–34*
        in cavities   32, *32*
        under tension   30–1, *30–2*
    one-handed, tied with the left hand   23–7, *24–7*
    reef   19, *20*
    slip   20, *20*
    surgeon's   30, *30*
    three-finger hitch   26, *27*
    triple throw   20, *20*
    two-handed   21–3, *21–3*
    using instruments   27–9, *28–9*
Kocher's arterial clamps   *12*
Kocher's toothed forceps   *10*

lachrymal duct repair   68
lactomer 9–1 thread   17
lag screw   139, *140*
laminaria tent   56
laparoscopy   180–3
laryngoscopes   60
laser   149
    in control of bleeding   157
Lawrence-type trocar and cannula   *47*
Lembert's stitch   40, 70, *71*
ligaments   120
ligatures   32–4, *33–4*, 155–6, *155*
liver   125–6, *126*
loupe   98, *98*
lumbar puncture   46
lung   127
lymph nodes   122–3

Mackintosh laryngoscope   49, *49*
Malecot catheter   *52*
malleable copper retractors   *12*
mattress stitches   39–40, 88
    everting   40
    inverting   40, 68, *69*
Mayo's needle-holder   *10*
mental attitude   1
minimal access   175–83
    acquiring skills   176–9
    closure   182–3
    diathermy in   182
    laparoscopy   180–3
    required skills   176
missiles, high-velocity   170
mucoperiosteum   122
muscle, skeletal   121–2
myocutaneous flaps   113–13, *113*
myotomy   76–7, *76*

needle biopsy   116–17, *117*
needle-holders   10–11, *10–11*
needles   34–9, *34–8*, 153
    curved, stitching with   37–9, *37–8*
    points   *36*
    round-bodied   36
    straight   34, *35*
neoplasms, dissection   152
nerves   120–1, *121*
neuropraxia   120
neurotmesis   121

obturator   44
ophthalmic needle-holder   *10*
oscillating diathermy   149
osteotome   131–2, *131–2*
ovarian tubes repair   68

packs   161–2, *161*
palpation   153
pancreas   126, *126*
pancreatic duct repair   68
parachute technique   72, *73*, 74, *75*, 96, *96*
Payr's lever-action intestinal clamps   *12*
peptic ulcer repair   68
percutaneous cannulation   84–5
    arteries   85
    veins   85

Related Titles...

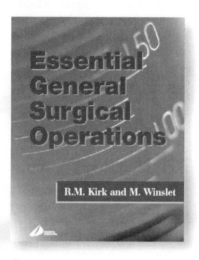

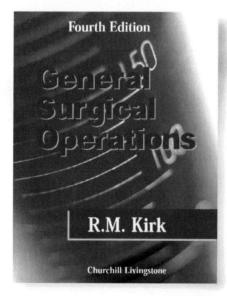

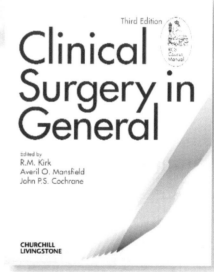

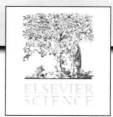